Dermatology

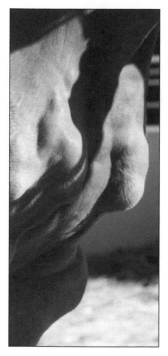

for the
Equine Practitioner

Dr. Ralf S. Mueller, Dr.med.vet.

Diplomate, American College of
Veterinary Dermatology

Fellow, Australian College of
Veterinary Scientists (Dermatology)

Diplomate, European College of
Veterinary Dermatology

Chief, Veterinary Allergy and
Dermatology Service

Medizinische Tierklinik,

Ludwig-Maximilians-University

Munich, Germany

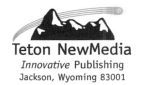

Teton NewMedia
Innovative Publishing
Jackson, Wyoming 83001

Executive Editor: Carroll C. Cann
Development Editor: Susan L. Hunsberger
Creative Director: Sue Haun 5640 Design, www.fiftysixforty.com
Production & Layout: Mike Albiniak 5640 Design, www.fiftysixforty.com

Teton NewMedia
P.O. Box 4833
Jackson, WY 83001
1-888-770-3165
www.tetonnm.com
www.veterinarywire.com

The authors and publisher have made every effort to provide an accurate reference text. However, they shall not be held responsible for problems arising from errors or omissions, or from misunderstandings on the part of the reader.

PRINTED IN THE UNITED STATES OF AMERICA

ISBN # 1-59161-023-0

Print number 5 4 3 2 1

Library of Congress Cataloging-in-Publication Data

Mueller, Ralf S.
    Dermatology for the equine practioner / Ralf S. Mueller.
      p. cm. – – (Made easy series)
    Includes bibliographical references and index.
    ISBN 1–59161–023–0
      1. Horses – – Diseases. 2. Veterinary dermatology. I. Title. II. Made easy series (Jackson Wyo.)

SF959.S54M84 2005
636.1'08965 – – dc22

                           2004063705

Dedication

This book is dedicated to Tony Stannard, my late mentor in equine dermatology and dermatopathology, an honest clinician of highest integrity who cared deeply about people and horses. Tony was able to simplify complicated scientific facts and mechanisms into easily understandable, practical essentials. Thank you, Tony!

Without the support and love of my wife, partner, and best friend Sonya Bettenay all my achievements including this book hardly would have been imaginable.

To all the colleagues whose support allowed me to develop the knowledge and experience that I hope will make this book useful in equine practice. Specific thanks to Drs. Andrea Cannon, Helen Power, Josie Traub-Dargatz and Linda Vogelnest for their suggestions on the manuscript and Drs. Hélène Amory, Luc Beco, Sonya Bettenay, John Cheney, Andrea Cannon, Gerhard Lösenbeck, Rod Rosychuk, Anthony Stannard, Josie Traub-Dargatz, Wayne Rosenkrantz and Sonja Zabel for some of the pictures. Ms. Amelie von Voigts-Rhetz provided some of the pictures of happy horses without skin disease.

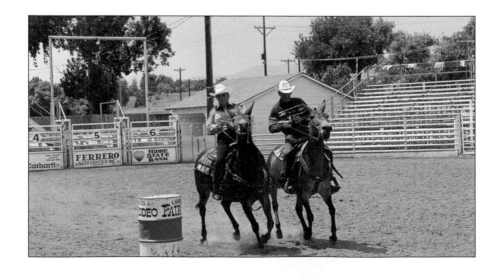

Preface

Dear Colleagues:

Horses are wonderful creatures that can teach us many life lessons. They are a source of admiration and pleasure for owners and veterinarians. Equine dermatology is an often underestimated part of equine practice. Due to the chronic nature of many skin problems they may cause frustration for veterinarians, clients, and patients alike. We have learned a lot about equine skin diseases in the last few years, but still have so much more to learn.

The goal of this book is to provide a practical approach to equine dermatology for the practitioner. There is information to help you diagnose and manage skin diseases seen every day in practice and enough detail for a solid workup in horses with rare or complicated skin diseases that may require further reading, advice from or referral to a veterinary dermatologist or equine internist.

Most of all, I hope it will allow you to enjoy your dermatology cases, to increase your diagnostic skills and improve the quality of life for your equine patients.

Warm regards

Ralf Mueller

Dr. med.vet. Dr.med.vet. habil. Ralf Mueller, MACVSc

Diplomate, American College of Veterinary Dermatology

Fellow, Australian College of Veterinary Scientists,

Diplomate, European College of Veterinary Dermatology

Table of Contents

Section 1 How To

Section 2 The Approach to Common Dermatologic Presentations

Section 3 Treatments

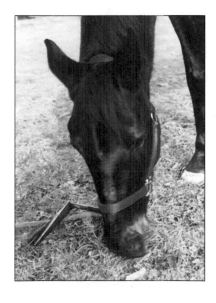

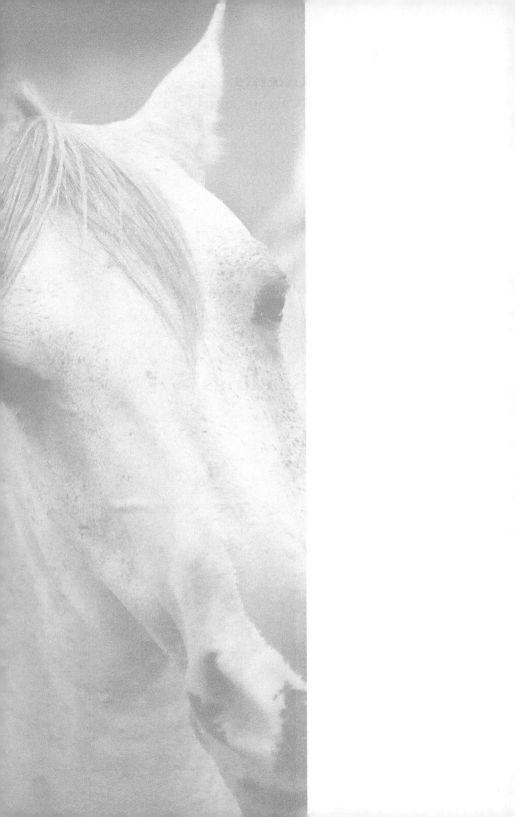

Section 1
"How To"

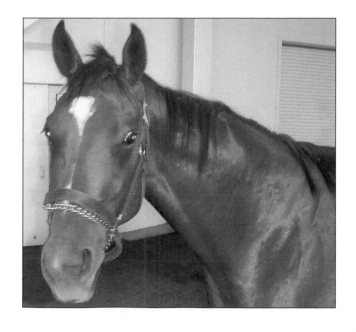

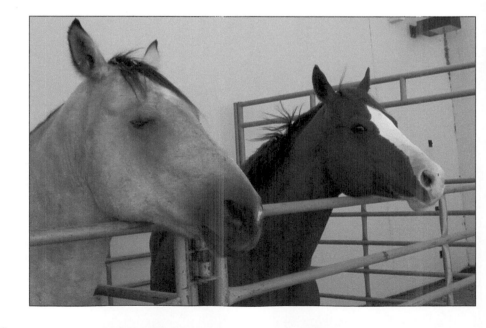

General Principles

The goal of this book is to provide a readily useable reference for equine dermatology with adequate information for a thorough and logical workup of a horse with skin disease. It also provides therapeutic protocols for the most common equine dermatologic problems. There are three sections in this book. The first covers how to take a dermatologic history, interpret the results of this history in light of the clinical findings, and which diagnostic tests to perform. The second explains an approach to common dermatologic presentations in equine practice. The last summarizes therapeutic options for specific conditions.

Some Helpful Hints

Scattered throughout the text, you will find the following symbols to help you focus on what is routine and what may be really important:

✓ This is a routine feature or basic point for understanding the subject discussed.

⚷ The key symbol will be used selectively to indicate a very important point to assist your understanding of the topic area.

✋ Stop. This does not look important, but it can really make a difference when trying to sort out unusual or difficult situations.

💣 Something serious will happen if you do not remember this, possibly resulting in injury or loss of the patient, and upset to the client.

In this section, I discuss key questions important in taking a dermatologic history for a horse. Specific dermatologic lesions are also discussed. Furthermore, I introduce various important diagnostic tests in equine dermatology, the necessary technique, and the interpretation of the results.

Dermatologic History

Clinical signs of various skin diseases are very similar and the etiology of a horse's skin disease may not be apparent based solely on clinical examination. The history will provide clues to the cause of the skin problem and allow prioritization of laboratory tests needed to confirm the diagnosis. I prefer my clients to complete a written questionnaire before or while I examine the horse to maximize and standardize the information to be gained from the history. We then review this questionnaire together. This decreases the time needed to obtain a good history and allows the owner to think about their horse's skin problem. A sample of a dermatology questionnaire is enclosed in the appendix. It is important to phrase questions appropriately because many owners leave out pertinent facts either because they are not aware of their relevance or because they think these facts may not be well received by the veterinarian. It may be necessary to ask the same question several times in different ways to obtain a meaningful answer. I cannot overemphasize the importance of taking a good and efficient dermatologic history, a skill which develops with experience, practice, and effective communication skills.

Question: *What is the breed of the patient?*

Relevance:

✓ Some breeds are predisposed to certain skin diseases and it can be worthwhile to keep a list of such breed predispositions within easy reach.

✓ Beware, breed predispositions may vary with geographic location!

✓ Arabians are predisposed to vascular hamartomas, and fading (pinky) syndrome.

✓ In Quarter horses, dermatosparaxis, linear keratosis/alopecia, leukotrichia, and unilateral papular dermatosis are more commonly seen.

✓ Mane and tail dystrophy occur more commonly in Appaloosas.

✓ Thoroughbreds, Quarterhorses, and Arabians may develop atopic dermatitis.

✓ Belgians are predisposed to epidermolysis bullosa, a disease recognized in foals.

Question: *How old was the horse when clinical signs were first recognized?*

Relevance:

✓ In foals, congenital and hereditary defects are more commonly seen. Pemphigus foliaceus may also occur in foals.

✓ Young adult horses are more commonly affected by atopic dermatitis, bacterial infections (trauma- or stress-induced), and dermatophytosis. Psoroptic mange is more commonly seen in young stabled horses.

✓ In middle age, immune-mediated skin diseases such as pemphigus foliaceus are seen more commonly.

✓ Older horses are more commonly affected by amyloidosis, Cushing's syndrome, and most neoplasias.

Question: *How long has the skin disease been present and how did it progress?*

Relevance:

✓ Acute onset of severe pruritus is typically associated with ectoparasite infestations such as scabies, psoroptic mange and trombiculidiasis, and with *Culicoides* hypersensitivity.

✓ If pruritus was the first sign and lesions occurred later, then atopic dermatitis, adverse food reaction, or ectoparasites should be considered. Pruritus and lesions that occur at the same time may be due to a wide variety of causes.

✓ Nonpruritic alopecia present for years without systemic signs points towards alopecia areata, follicular dysplasia, or hereditary alopecia.

✓ Chronic wounds with or without draining tracts necessitate the search for an infectious organism.

Question: *Is the horse pruritic?*

Relevance:

✓ Pruritus in horses can be difficult to identify. Owners often do not consider rubbing, stomping, or biting as clinical signs of pruritus.

Careful questioning may be needed to identify pruritus in some patients.

✔ The presence of pruritus with skin lesions is not of diagnostic value, given that many skin diseases cause pruritus. However, pruritus without lesions typically indicates allergic skin diseases or ectoparasite infestations.

✔ The perceived severity of pruritus may vary with the owner. Some owners deny the presence of pruritus despite watching their horse rub or bite during a clinical examination. Others will be astute and accurate observers. Good communication skills and judgment are essential to form a realistic opinion of the degree of pruritus.

Question: *Is the disease seasonal?*

Relevance:

✔ In temperate climates, insect bite hypersensitivities frequently cause disease in spring, summer, and/or fall. Whether clinical signs are absent or milder in the colder season depends on specific environmental conditions.

✔ Atopic dermatitis may also be seasonal in certain climates. In many temperate climates it may be more noticeable in spring and summer if caused by tree and grass pollens or worsen in summer and autumn because of weed pollens. Tropical or subtropical climates usually have an extended pollen season. Hypersensitivities to grain mill dust or storage mites in stabled horses are often nonseasonal.

✔ Many horses with atopic dermatitis or insect bite hypersensitivity are affected more severely and for longer periods each year as they age.

Question: *Is the horse systemically ill?*

Relevance:

✔ Sneezing and coughing may be seen concurrently with atopic dermatitis and caused by airborne allergies.

✔ Pulmonary edema may be seen in sick horses with purpura hemorrhagica.

✔ Fever and depression may be seen with viral diseases, vasculitis, granulomatous disease, lymphosarcoma, or systemic lupus erythematosis (SLE)-like disease.

Question: *What is the horse's diet?*

Relevance:

✓ Knowing all dietary ingredients is necessary to formulate a diet trial.

✓ If a diet was fed in the past and it was not a true elimination diet, was not fed exclusively, or not fed for an appropriate length of time, a diet trial will need to be repeated.

☞ Contrary to common belief, adverse food reactions typically do not occur immediately after a change in diet.

✋ Remember to ask about vitamins and other supplements, which are often forgotten, when diet is discussed with the client.

Question: *Do other horses have regular contact with the patient or share tack or grooming equipment? Do they show cutaneous signs?*

Relevance:

✓ If other horses are similarly affected, contagious diseases such as dermatophytosis or ectoparasites are more likely.

✋ Other animals may serve as a reservoir for ectoparasites without themselves showing clinical signs.

Question: *Was the disease treated before? If so, what medications were used and how successful was the treatment? This question needs to address both what veterinarians prescribed and what the owner/handler used from their own "pharmacy."*

Relevance:

Response to previous therapy can be of tremendous value in the diagnostic evaluation of skin disease.

✓ Initial response to glucocorticoid administration is not necessarily helpful because many skin diseases improve for a short period with this symptomatic, non-specific treatment.

✓ Repeated substantial response to low-dose glucocorticoid therapy suggests hypersensitivities. However, lack of response does not rule out hypersensitivity.

✓ Repeated response to antibiotics and glucocorticoids given in combination is of little help.

✋ It is essential to ask how much the horse improved while receiving medication as owners tend to judge a treatment as not helpful if it did not completely cure the disease.

🖐 Horse owners often use home-made remedies or left-over medications without specific mention and need to be questioned specifically in this regard.

Question: *When was the last medication given?*

Relevance:

Recent administration of medication may affect the clinical presentation.

✔ Long-term glucocorticoid therapy (systemic or topical) may affect the results of allergy tests - both intradermal testing and serum testing for allergen-specific IgE. It may also affect histopathologic findings and clinical pathologic results.

✔ Antihistamines will influence intradermal testing.

✔ Remember to ask specifically for deworming or vitamin supplements, which are also forms of pharmacotherapy.

Question: *Does the horse get better with a change in environment (other paddock, stabling, etc.)?*

Relevance:

✔ Improvement in another environment suggests involvement of an environmental allergen, irritant, or insect-bite hypersensitivity.

✔ Lack of improvement does not rule out these airborne and contact allergens as they may be the same in different locations.

Question: *What is the current deworming protocol and what insect control is used?*

Relevance:

✔ Regular appropriate use of ivermectin for deworming decreases the likelihood of diseases such as onchocerciasis and oxyuridiasis.

✔ Regular insect control does not necessarily rule out insect bite hypersensitivity.

Dermatologic Examination

A dermatologic examination requires adequate lighting, a systematic and thorough approach, and should always include a general physical examination. Observation from a distance should be followed by close inspection of skin and mucous membranes. Start at the head, inspect the lips, mouth, eyes, ears visually, but also use your hands to evaluate the neck and the trunk; examine the hairs and skin of mane and tail, lift up the tail to inspect the perianal area, and then each leg to inspect the frog and sole of each hoof.

General Observation

Localized or Generalized problems

✓ If the skin lesions are focal, and localized to one area, consider an infectious cause such as for example pythiosis, phaeohyphomycosis, or pseudomycetoma due to dermatophytes.

✓ Cutaneous neoplastic diseases are typically localized, at least initially.

✓ Generalized disorders are more commonly due to hypersensitivities or systemic conditions such as immune-mediated skin diseases.

Symmetry

Systemic disorders such as allergies or pemphigus foliaceus typically cause bilaterally symmetric lesions.

Asymmetric lesions more commonly have external causes such as dermatophilosis or dermatophytosis.

Haircoat Quality, Color, and Shine

✓ Is the haircoat dull or shiny? A dull haircoat may be due to primary metabolic disease, external parasites, nutritional deficiencies, or may develop with chronic skin disease.

✓ Are there coat or mane/tail color changes and if so, did they develop with initial skin lesions or after those lesions had been present for a while. Hair color changes can be the consequence of chronic or severe inflammation or a primary disorder.

✓ Changes in the hair quality (either to a coarse coat or to a fine coat) are suggestive of hormonal disease or follicular dysplasia.

After a general examination begins a detailed inspection of the skin and mucous membranes. Special attention should be paid to individual lesions. Try to differentiate primary from secondary lesions. Primary lesions are initial eruptions caused directly by the underlying disease process. Secondary lesions evolve from primary lesions or are caused by the horse (self-trauma) or environment (medications). Differentiating primary from secondary lesions is important to understand the underlying pathomechanism and to formulate a relevant list of differential diagnoses.

Primary Lesions

Macule

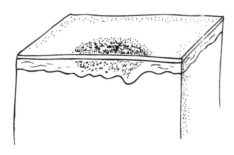

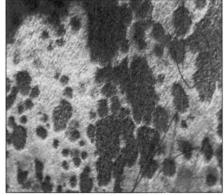

Figure 1-1A

Definition: A focal, circumscribed, nonpalpable change in color up to 1 cm in diameter. (A lesion > 1cm is termed a patch.)

Pathogenesis: Pigmentation change due to decreased or increased melanin production, erythema due to inflammation, or local hemorrhage due to trauma or vasculitis.

Figure 1-1B

Differential diagnoses - depigmentation: Vitiligo, "Lupus erythematosus-like syndrome," Arabian fading syndrome.

Differential diagnosis -erythema: Inflammation due to a variety of underlying diseases (blanches with diascopy, when a slide is pressed onto the erythematosus lesion) or hemorrhage due to vasculopathies or coagulopathies (does not blanch on diascopy).

Papule

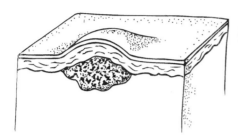

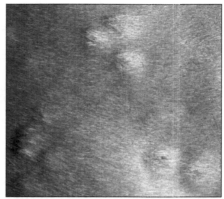

Figure 1-2A
Definition: A solid elevation of up to 1 cm in diameter. Larger lesions are called *plaques*.
Pathogenesis: Influx of inflammatory cells into the dermis, focal epidermal hyperplasia, early neoplastic lesions.

Figure 1-2B
Differential diagnosis: Bacterial folliculitis, fungal folliculitis, *Culicoides* hypersensitivity, scabies, contact allergy, erythema multiforme, drug eruption.

Pustule

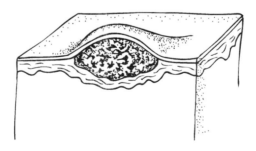

Figure 1-3
Definition: A small circumscribed area within the epidermis filled with pus.
Pathogenesis: Most pustules are filled with neutrophils, but eosinophilic pustules may also be seen. Aspiration cytology and biopsy are indicated. Pustules are very rarely seen in horses.
Differential diagnoses: Bacterial infection, fungal infection, immune-mediated skin disease.

Vesicle

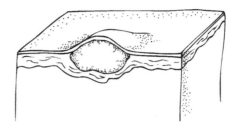

Figure 1-4
Definition: A small circumscribed area within or below the epidermis filled with clear fluid. Larger vesicles are called *bullae*. Vesicles are very fragile and thus transient.
Pathogenesis: Spongiosis and extracellular fluid collection due to inflammation and loss of intercellular cohesion. Vesicles are very rarely seen in horses.
Differential diagnoses: Autoimmune and congenital skin diseases, viral diseases, or irritant dermatitis.

Wheal

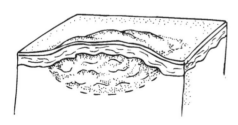

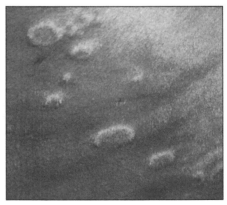

Figure 1-5A Wheal
Definition: A sharply circumscribed, raised, edematous and transient lesion. Individual wheals may be present for only minutes to hourse, but if the stimulus causing wheal formation persists, wheals will continue to be observed.

Pathogenesis: Cutaneous edema.

Figure 1-5B Urticarial wheals
Differential diagnoses: All hypersensitivities such as insect bite hypersensitivity, atopic dermatitis and food reaction, drug eruption.

Nodule

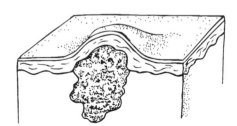

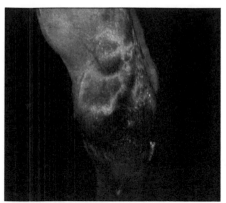

Figure 1-6A Nodule
Definition: A circumscribed, solid
elevation > 1 cm in diameter that
extends into deeper layers of the skin.
Pathogenesis: Infiltration of inflammatory or neoplastic cells, deposition of
fibrin or crystalline material into the
dermis and subcutis.

Figure 1-6B Nodule
Differential diagnoses: Eosinophilic
granuloma, deep bacterial or fungal
infections, neoplastic diseases.

Tumor

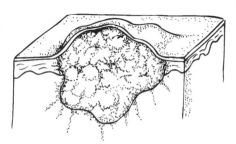

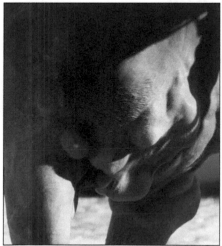

Figure 1-7A Tumor
Definition: A large mass involving skin
or subcutaneous tissue.
Pathogenesis: Massive influx of inflammatory or neoplastic cells.

Figure 1-7B Tumor
Differential diagnoses:
Granulomatous diseases of sterile,
bacterial or fungal origin, neoplastic
diseases.

Primary or Secondary Lesions
Alopecia

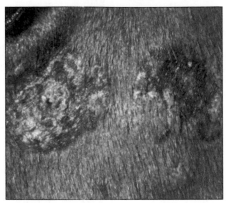

Figure 1-8 Alopecia
Definition: Loss of hair can be partial or complete, inflammatory or noninflammatory.
Pathogenesis: Self-trauma, damage to the hair or hair follicle due to dysplasia, inflammation and/or infection.
Differential diagnoses: Primary lesion in alopecia areata, follicular dysplasias, telogen effluvium, anagen defluxion. Secondary lesion in pruritic skin diseases, bacterial or fungal folliculitis.

Scale

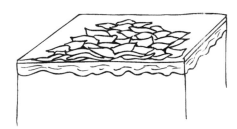

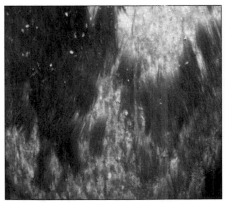

Figure 1-9A Scale
Definition: An accumulation of loose fragments of the horny layer of the skin.

Pathogenesis: Either increased production of keratinocytes (such as in disorders of keratinization) or increased retention. Scales are very common in horses.

Figure 1-9B Scale
Differential diagnoses: Primary lesion in follicular dysplasias, idiopathic seborrheas. Secondary lesion in diseases associated with chronic skin inflammation.

Crust

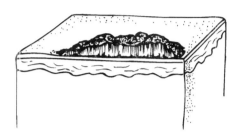

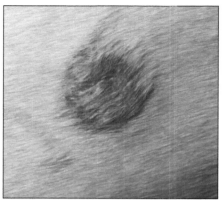

Figure 1-10A Crust
Definition: Adherence of exudate, serum, pus, blood, scales or medications to the skin surface.

Figure 1-10B Crust
Differential diagnoses: Secondary lesion in a variety of skin diseases such as dermatophytosis, dermatophilosis, pemphigus foliaceus.

Secondary Lesions

Epidermal Collarettes

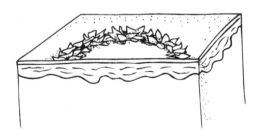

Figure 1-11 Epidermal collarette
Definition: Circular lesions with loose keratin flakes or "peeling" keratin arranged in a circle.
Pathogenesis: Remnant of a pustule or vesicle after the top part (the "roof") has been lost.
Differential diagnoses: Bacterial or fungal infection, immune-mediated skin disease.

Erosion

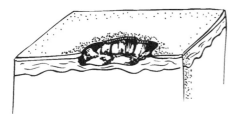

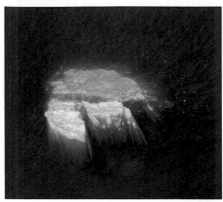

Figure 1-12A Erosion
Definition: A shallow epidermal defect that does not breach the dermo-epidermal junction.
Pathogenesis: Trauma or inflammation leads to rapid death and/or loss of keratinocytes.

Figure 1-12B Erosion
Differential diagnoses: Skin diseases associated with self trauma such as infections or allergies.

Ulcer

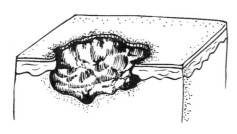

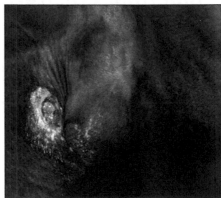

Figure 1-13A Ulcer
Definition: Focal loss of epidermis with exposure of underlying dermis.
Pathogenesis: More severe trauma and/or deep and severe inflammation, genetic or immune-mediated diseases damaging the dermo-epidermal junction such as epidermolysis bullosa or bullous pemphigoid.

Figure 1-13B Ulcer
Differential diagnoses: Pruritic skin diseases leading to self trauma and diseases that affect the dermoepidermal junction.

Diagnostic Tests Useful in Equine Dermatology

Cytology

Indications

Skin surface cytology is always a useful step in the evaluation of a horse with skin disease. It is particularly helpful in any pruritic, scaly, odoriferous, or alopecic horse in which bacterial or fungal infection is a differential diagnosis. Cytologic samples are obtained by a variety of methods such as skin scrapings, aspirations, touch impressions, ear swabs, and tape preparations.

✓ A superficial skin scraping is used when the skin is slightly moist or greasy.

✓ An aspirated sample is useful for the evaluation of pustular content and intradermal or subcutaneous nodules.

✓ An impression smear is used to obtain samples from moist or oily skin, or oozing or discharging lesions.

✓ Dry scaly skin is evaluated by tape preparations.

Technique

1. Skin scraping for cytology

✓ Affected skin is exposed and the surface of the skin scraped very gently and superficially with a scalpel blade in the direction of hair growth. The skin should not be abraded during the scraping. An area of 2 x 2 cm should be scraped.

✓ The debris collected on the blade is applied to a slide and spread with the blade in a "buttering the bread" motion (Figure 1-14).

👋 In contrast to skin scrapings for the detection of ectoparasites, no mineral oil is used in skin scrapings for cytology.

2. Fine needle aspiration of nodules

✓ Aspiration of nodules or abscesses is undertaken with a 12-ml syringe and a 22-ga (or with more vascular tissue a 25-ga) needle.

✓ The skin should be disinfected gently using an alcohol swab before sampling.

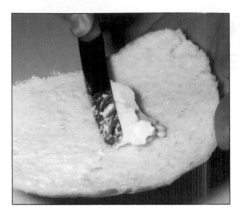

Figure 1-14 Debris collected with a skin scraping is spread onto a slide with a "butter the bread" motion.

✓ The needle is inserted with the syringe attached and aspirated several times (up to the 5-10 ml mark if possible).

✓ Before the syringe with needle is removed, the plunger needs to be released to release pressure.

✓ It is important to release the pressure before withdrawal of the needle or the aspirate can be sucked back into the barrel of the syringe, from which it may not be retrieved.

✓ Alternatively, a needle may be inserted without attached syringe, reoriented several times within the nodules and then withdrawn.

✓ The needle is detached, the plunger pulled back, and the needle reattached.

✓ Cells or exudate are then blown onto a slide. The smear is air dried.

3. Impression smear

✓ In horses with moist or greasy skin, the slide can be rubbed or impressed directly onto affected skin (Figure 1-15).

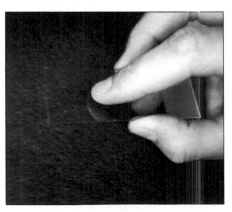

Figure 1-15 Impression smears are obtained by gently pressing a slide onto affected skin.

4. Tape preparation

✔ A direct impression technique uses clear sticky tape to collect debris from the surface of the skin. Although quick, this method requires practice to establish what is "normal."

✔ The sticky side of the tape is pressed onto the skin (Figure 1-16).

Figure 1-16 The tape is pressed sticky-side down onto affected skin.

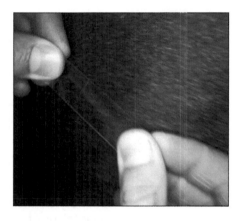

✔ The tape is then mounted onto a slide (also sticky side down) onto a drop of methylene blue or the blue stain of DiffQuick (Figure 1-17).

Figure 1-17 Tape is then pressed sticky-side down onto a drop of methylene blue on a slide.

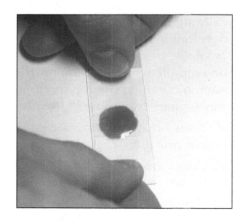

✔ The tape/slide is then evaluated microscopically. If needed, immersion oil can be used on the tape for 1000 x magnification.

✔ Items of interest that can be identified include inflammatory cells such as neutrophils (which may have exocytosed through the epidermis in response to a superficial infection), yeast, bacteria such as cocci or rods, eosinophils, and macrophages (Figures 1-18 and 1-19). Nucleated epithelial cells reflect a keratinization abnormality.

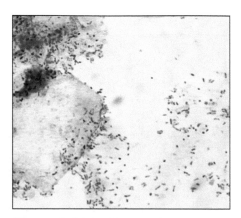 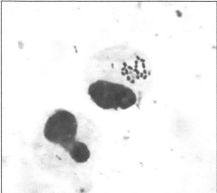

Figure 1-18 (Left) Keratinocytes, bacteria (pink to dark purple) and melanosomes (black) on cytology of a horse.
Figure 1-19 (Right) Neutrophil with intracellular cocci.

Interpretation

🖐 Evaluation of cytology obtained by any of the techniques described above requires practice to differentiate normal from clinically significant changes. Now would be a great time to begin developing the skills needed, if you don't feel comfortable with cytologic evaluations already. If you are inexperienced, sending in one sample while holding onto the other and evaluating it after having obtained the report from the clinical pathologist is a good way to start "supervised" learning.

✔ Yeast organisms are not commonly found in horses, but cause severe pruritus occasionally.

✔ Cocci are most often *Staphylococcus* spp., rods such as Corynebacteria may be found in some patients.

🖐 The number of organisms is important. Occasional cocci or yeast are probably not relevant. Don't mistake exogenous bacterial contaminants for infection.

✔ Inflammatory cells with intracellular organisms are pathognomonic for a clinically relevant infection.

✔ Eosinophils typically indicate allergic or parasitic skin disease.

✿✲ Neoplastic cells may be difficult to recognize so confirmation by a clinical pathologist is appropriate. Neoplastic lesions of the skin should not be diagnosed by cytology exclusively; a biopsy should always confirm the clinical and cytological suspicions.

✔ Acantholytic cells are keratinocytes that have lost their intercellular connections (the desmosomes) and appear as round cells with a purple cytoplasm and a central, dark purple nucleus. These cells suggest pemphigus foliaceus. A biopsy is indicated to confirm the diagnosis.

☙➼ Remember that superficial bacterial and yeast infections are usually secondary to other diseases which need to be identified and treated to manage the horse's skin disease entirely.

☙➼ Cytologic re-evaluation at the end of antimicrobial therapy is crucial to evaluate success of therapy.

Dermatophilosis preparation

✔ Remove crusts and clip excess hair of these samples.

✔ Place crusts in saline on a clean slide.

✔ Crush material and allow to air dry.

✔ Heat fix to the point where slide is just too warm for the skin on the back of your hand.

✔ Typically dermatophilus organisms have a "railroad-track appearance" (Figures 1-20 and 1-21). However, this classic presentation is not always seen. Any clumped cocci should be evaluated further.

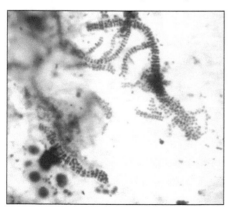 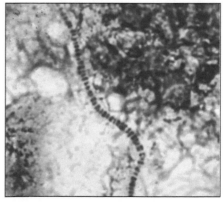

Figure 1-20 (Left) Dermatophilus organisms on cytology. Diffquick, x 1000. (Courtesy of Dr. Rod Rosychuk.)

Figure 1-21 (Right) Dermatophilus congolensis organisms on cytology, note the "railroad track" appearance. DiffQuick, x 1000. (Courtesy of Dr. Rod Rosychuk.)

Superficial Skin Scrapings

Indications

Ectoparasitism should be considered in any pruritic, scaly, or crusty horse. Skin scrapings to check for *Psoroptes* spp., *Chorioptes* spp., *Scabies scabiei*, *Dermanyssus gallinae*, or lice should be performed.

Technique

✓ If *Chorioptes equi* is suspected, preferred areas for scrapings are the pastern and palmar cannon regions. For *Psoroptes* spp., samples of ear wax (*P. hippotis*) or skin scrapings (*P. equi*) should be evaluated.

✓ The hair should be removed by gently clipping with #40 clipper blades. Mites may be difficult to find. The bigger the surface area scraped, the greater will be the chance of a positive skin scraping.

✓ To facilitate the process, spread a thin layer of mineral oil on the clipped skin (Figure 1-22).

✓ Then scrape the oil off the skin with a #11 scalpel blade (Figure 1-23) and transfer the removed material to one or more glass slides (Figure 1-24). Additional oil may need to be added on to the slide to evenly mix and disperse the sample.

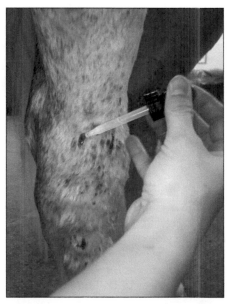

Figure 1-22 Mineral or paraffin oil is applied onto affected skin.

✔ A cover slip is used to allow rapid yet thorough evaluation of collected debris and the slide(s) is(are) evaluated under low power (40 or 100). To ensure the evaluation of all the sample, follow a systemic regime such as from the left upper corner to the right lower corner.

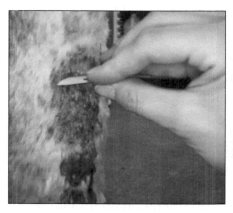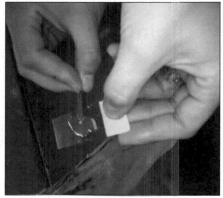

Figure 1-23 (Left) A scalpel blade is used to scrape applied oil off the affected and clipped skin...

Figure 1-24 (Right) ...and the oil and gathered debris are transferred to a slide.

Interpretation

The finding of any mites or eggs of *Sarcoptes, Psorioptes*, or *Chorioptes* spp., *Trombicula autumnalis, Dermanyssus gallinae*, or lice such as *Damalinia equi* or *Haematobinus asini* is diagnostic (Figures 1-25 and 1-26). Negative scrapings do not rule out the presence of mites and clinical disease. Response to a therapeutic trial for the suspected ectoparasite may be necessary.

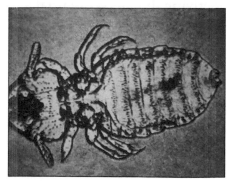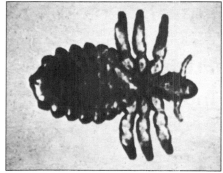

Figure 1-25 An equine biting louse, *Damalinia equi.*
(Courtesy of Dr. John Cheney.)

Figure 1-26 An equine sucking louse, *Hematobinus asini.*
(Courtesy of Dr. John Cheney.)

Deep Skin Scrapings

Indications

Demodicosis is rare in the horse and typically secondary to systemic disease, but any horse with patchy alopecia and/or papules should be scraped for the presence of *D. caballi* (face) or *D. equi* (trunk).

Technique

✔ Because *Demodex* mites live deep in the hair follicle, it may be useful to squeeze the skin as hard as the horse will tolerate in an attempt to push mites out from the depths of the follicles before scraping.

✔ A blade covered with mineral oil is stroked in the direction of hair growth *until capillary bleeding* is observed.

✔ Lesions on the face may be difficult to scrape. An alternative method to assess for *Demodex* mites is to pluck hair from suspicious lesions. The hair is placed in a drop of mineral oil on a slide. A cover slip is placed on top, and the hair roots are evaluated microscopically for the presence of mites.

✔ The finding of more than one mite should be considered diagnostic. If you find one mite, scrapings should be repeated to determine if this is of clinical significance (in which case more mites should be found on subsequent scrapings).

Interpretation

It is important to assess *and to note* the site of scraping, the relative numbers of adults, larvae/nymphs and eggs per low power field (LPF). Equine demodicosis usually occurs due to primary systemic diseases, search for an underlying disease is essential and treatment of such underlying disease more important than treatment of equine demodicosis.

Fungal Culture

Indications

A dermatophyte culture may be indicated in any horse with possible dermatophyte infection and thus in any patient with alopecia, papules, pustules, scales and/or crusts.

Technique

✓ Hairs and scale from the edge of a lesion should be taken (Figure 1-29).

Figure 1-29 Hairs and scales from the edge of skin lesions are chosen for fungal culture.

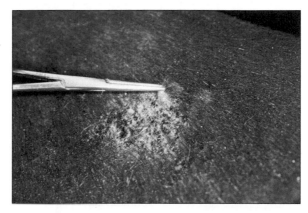

✓ Sabouraud's agar is the most common medium for fungal cultures. However, as a diagnostic aid most practitioners use dermatophyte test medium (DTM) (Figure 1-30). DTM is a Sabouraud agar with a color indicator and added ingredients to inhibit growth of saprophytes and bacteria. Niacin (or more readily available a couple of drops of vitamin B complex solution) should be added to the culture medium for optimal growth conditions for *Trichophyton equinum* var. *equinum*, but is not needed for *T. equinum* var. *autotrophicum*.

✓ After being innoculated, the culture jars should be incubated at between 25° and 30° C at 30% humidity, or in a warm, dark corner with the *lids* **not** *screwed down* tightly.

✓ Cultures should be incubated for 2 to 3 weeks and must be evaluated daily.

Figure 1-30
A culture on dermatophyte test medium taken from a horse.

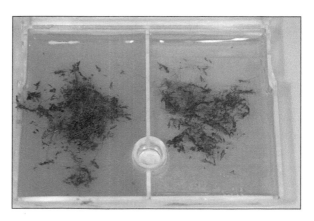

Interpretation

A pH change (and subsequently color change) that occurs **as the colony is growing** indicates dermatophyte growth (Figures 1-31, 1-32 and 1-33). These fungi use protein preferentially producing alkaline metabolites, which cause the pH and color change. It is imperative that the color change is observed coincidentally with the development of the colony as color changes may also occur in association with mature (i.e., large) saprophyte colonies.

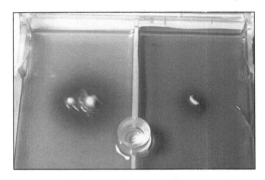

Figure 1-31 A positive dermatophyte culture with early color change of the dermatophyte test medium.

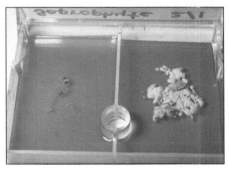 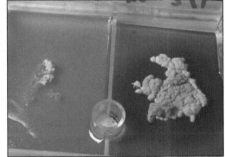

Figure 1-32 (Left) A saprophyte culture initially grows without color change...
Figure 1-33 (Right) ....and then the grown culture changes the medium color rapidly.

Saprophytes initially utilize carbohydrates, which are not associated with a color change. Only after all carbohydrates have been used and the colony has already grown, do they utilize proteins and change the color and pH of the medium. It may be impossible to distinguish on gross appearance whether a mature colony with significant red pigmentation to the underlying and surrounding agar is a pathogenic or saprophytic fungus. Therefore daily evaluation of fungal colonies is essential.

✓ Always check the colony microscopically. Clear sticky tape is impressed gently onto the culture (sticky side down), then laid onto a drop of methylene blue or the blue stain of DiffQuick (also sticky side down) on a microscope slide and evaluated under the microscope. The surface of the sticky tape acts as its own cover slip. If required, microscope oil can be placed directly onto the surface of the tape. If you do not have the time or skill to complete this identification, submit the DTM culture to a diagnostic laboratory for speciation. This will give clues to the source of the dermatophyte and its zoonotic potential.

✓ *T. equinum* grows as a flat colony with a white to cream-colored, powdery surface and a deep yellow pigment can be visualized on the back of the colony (reverse pigment) (Figures 1-34 and 1-35). Stalked microconidia are seen microscopically, macroconidia are less common (Figure 1-36).

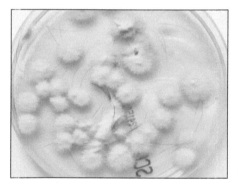 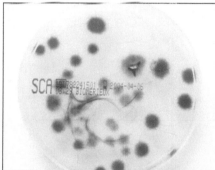

Figure 1-34 (Left) *Trichophyton equinum*, culture. (Courtesy of Dr. Gerhard Lösenbeck.)

Figure 1-35 (Right) *Trichophyton equinum* culture seen from the bottom, note the yellow-to-brown reverse pigment. (Courtesy of Dr. Gerhard Lösenbeck.)

Figure 1-36 *Trichophyton equinum*, note the numerous microconidia and the few macroconidia. (Courtesy of Dr. Gerhard Lösenbeck.)

✓ *T. verrucosum* has macroscopic features similar to *T. equinum*, but the reverse pigment is typically tan to brown. Additional distinguishing features are microconidia attached singly or in grapelike clusters along the hyphae, and less commonly cigar-shaped, thin-walled macroconidia.

✓ *Microsporum canis* grows as a white, wooly colony with a yellowish reverse pigment (which may be difficult to assess if grown on DTM). Abundant spindle-shaped macroconidia with knobs at the terminal ends and typically more than six internal compartments are seen microscopically (Figure 1-37).

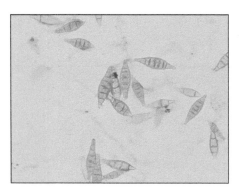

Figure 1-37 *Microsporum canis,* note the numerous macroconidia. (Courtesy of Dr. Gerhard Lösenbeck.)

✓ M. *canis* is a zoophilic dermatophyte and horses typically were infected by another animal or human. Humans and other animals in contact with the patient are at risk to develop the infection or may be asymptomatic carriers and need to be carefully evaluated and possibly treated as well.

✓ M. *gypseum* has a granular, beige culture with yellowish reverse pigment and has thin-walled macroconidia with fewer than six internal compartments. M. gypseum is a geophilic fungus that is acquired by exposure to contaminated soil and thus has a lower zoonotic potential.

✓ *Trichophyton mentagrophytes* grows in variable (powdery versus fluffy etc) colonies that characteristically have a few, cigar-shaped macroconidia and globous microconidia. Typical hosts for *T. mentagrophytes* are rodents; infections are usually associated with exposure to these hosts or their immediate environment.

Trichogram

Indication

Trichograms may be useful in any alopecic animal as well as in animals with suspected dermatophytosis and associated papules, pustules, or crusting.

Technique

✓ A forceps is used to forcefully pluck hairs from affected skin.

✓ The hairs are then placed onto a slide and evaluated under low power. I generally use mineral oil and a cover slip to prevent the hair sample blowing all over the table rather than remaining under the microscope.

Interpretation

A trichogram is taken for several possible reasons:

✓ Does a horse create hair loss by rubbing or does the hair fall out for other reasons? If the animal is pruritic and rubs the hair off, the tips of the hairs are broken off. Any trauma to the hair shaft such as occurs in dermatophytosis may also cause hair with broken ends. If the hair falls out for other reasons, the tips are tapered.

✓ Trichograms may also be used to diagnose equine demodicosis. If mites are found microscopically, the diagnosis is confirmed. If however no mites are present, demodicosis cannot be ruled out!

✓ Fungal spores or hyphae may be seen on hair shafts of horses with dermatophytosis. A normal trichogram however does not rule out dermatophytosis.

Biopsy

Indication

✓ Any skin disorder that appears **unusual** to the clinician should be biopsied.

✓ A biopsy should also be considered if lesions **fail to respond** to appropriate empiric therapy.

✓ **Nodules** may be neoplastic and should be biopsied.

✓ Any suspected disease for which treatment is **expensive and/or life-threatening** should be confirmed histopathologically.

✓ Finally, one of the best reasons to perform a skin biopsy is to rule out other diagnoses. I think this is an allergy but... In such a situation, the biopsy report of chronic hyperplastic dermatitis with mononuclear and/or eosinophilic perivascular infiltrate is consistent with this and other dermatoses have been eliminated. A supportive pathologic diagnosis interpreted in conjunction with the clinical impressions may be just as useful as a confirmatory diagnosis.

✓ More quiescent forms of equine sarcoid may react to sampling by rapid growth and expansion, the need for histopathological confirmation has to be carefully weighed against this risk and a decision made for each individual horse based on site of the lesion, differential diagnoses and discussions with the owner prior to the procedure.

Biopsy Technique

Site Selection

✓ Selection of the site requires careful examination of the entire horse for the most representative samples, identification of the primary and secondary lesions present and the formation of a list of differential diagnoses before biopsy.

✋ With the exception of a solitary nodule it is recommended that *multiple tissue samples* should be taken. These should include primary lesions if present, contain a representative range of lesions, and should be taken and handled carefully. A normal sample of haired skin should also be included.

✓ *Depigmenting* lesions should be biopsied in an area of *active depigmentation* (gray color) rather than the final stage (white or pink color).

✓ *Alopecia* should be biopsied in the center of the worst area as well as in junctional and normal areas. A suture through the subcutaneous fat may be used to identify for the pathologist where a particular sample was taken.

✓ Ulcers and erosions are typically non-rewarding sites to biopsy. Histopathology will reveal just that, an ulcer, and is thus not helpful for the diagnosis.

Preparation of the Site

✓ Do not prepare in any way the skin surface prior to a biopsy procedure. Even topical application and air drying of alcohol may alter the epidermis. Infection as a result of lack of surgical preparation is a very rare complication.

✓ If crusts are present, take care to leave these on the skin. If they are accidentally dislodged they should still be placed in the formalin. A note "please cut in crusts" should be added to the pathology request form. Crusts may contain diagnostic information such as microorganisms or acantholytic cells.

Wedge versus Punch Biopsy

✓ There are two commonly employed biopsy techniques in veterinary medicine, the *punch biopsy* and the *wedge biopsy*. The latter is commonly employed as an excisional technique when removing solitary nodules. Wedge biopsy technique is also indicated for vesicular lesions (which could be ruptured with a punch biopsy procedure), suspected cases of panniculitis (if sufficient depth of biopsy cannot be achieved with a punch) or when biopsying the edge of a lesion in a spindle shape (which allows correct orientation of the lesion in the laboratory where spindle-shaped lesions are always cut in longitudinally).

✓ The *punch biopsy* is easier to use, requires less instrumentation, is quicker and the biopsy method of choice for suspected infectious, inflammatory, and endocrine dermatoses. Disposable biopsy punches are readily available and a diameter of 8 mm should be used.

✓ Overlying hair needs to be clipped and gently removed and the biopsy site is marked with a water-proof marker pen (Figure 1-38). If crusts are present it may be less traumatic to use scissors.

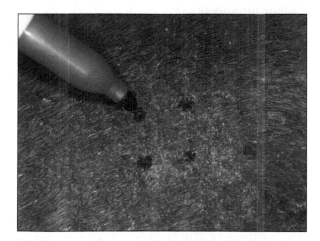

Figure 1-38 The biopsy site is gently clipped and marked with a water-proof marker pen.

🖐 Depending on the location of the biopsy sites, concurrent systemic sedation in addition to local anesthesia may be needed, particularly if specimens are taken from the face, limbs and/or ventrum! The biopsy sites are anesthesized by the subcutaneous injection of 1-ml xylocaine (or the less stinging prilocaine) (Figure 1-39). Infiltrate below the site from outside to minimize any artificial disruption of the sample.

☟ Allow 3 to 5 minutes for the local anesthetic to have effect.

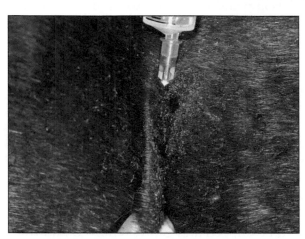

Figure 1-39 Local anaesthetic is injected subcutaneously.

✔ Punch biopsy is performed by using the punch at right angles to the surface of the skin and placed over the selected lesion. Apply firm continuous pressure and rotate the punch in one direction (note carefully!) until you feel the punch slide into the subcutaneous fat (Figure 1-40). A clue that you are completely through the skin is that blood will well up around the biopsy.

✔ The section of tissue is grasped at the base by the subcutaneous fat (Figure 1-41) and subcutaneous attachments severed. Under no circumstances should the dermis or epidermis be grasped with forceps because this leads to crush artifact. Crushed tissue may be misinterpreted as scarring at best and at worst renders the sample worthless. Using small instruments such as an ophthalmic rat tooth forceps will facilitate the biopsy procedure. The tissue is rolled on gauze to gently blot blood.

✔ The unit of tissue and cardboard is placed in 10% formalin (tissue side down) and allowed to fix for several hours before sectioning. The volume of formalin required is at least 10 times the volume of the sample. Nodules should be sectioned into 1-cm thick pieces to allow adequate penetration of the formalin into the center of the lesion.

Figure 1-40 The punch is placed vertically onto the surface and rotated in only one direction.

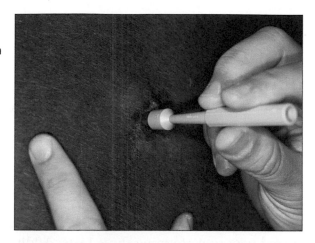

Figure 1-41 The sample is removed by grabbing its base with a forceps and cutting it.

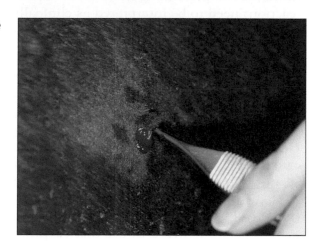

Submission of Biopsy Samples

✓ Equally as important to choosing appropriate biopsy sites and obtaining adequate numbers of samples is providing the pathologist with a complete, detailed history and clinical description. Careful completion of an appropriate skin biopsy request form will greatly improve the chances of a diagnostic report.

A differential diagnosis list is important with any clinical case and is essential with dermatologic patients. This list is important for the clinician to ensure that he or she has considered all options and obtained as much information from the owner as possible and necessary before taking the biopsy. It is also essential for the pathologist and to aid in choosing if additional tests or stains are needed to rule out or confirm unusual diseases.

Serum Testing for Allergen-Specific IgE

Indication

The diagnosis of atopy is a diagnosis of exclusion after all other causes of pruritus have been considered and ruled out by diagnostic steps. Probable environmental allergens can be further defined by serum or intradermal testing, if an owner of an atopic horse is either curious what causes the problem or interested in allergen-specific immunotherapy. Most nonallergic horses will show some positive reactions to both intradermal testing and serum testing for allergen-specific IgE. It is essential, that atopic dermatitis is diagnosed *prior* to performing these tests. Additionally the positive reactions need to be interpreted as clinically significant or not based on the horse's environmental exposures.

Interpretation

✓ Measurement for equine allergen-specific IgE is available from a number of commercial laboratories. Laboratory techniques have improved over the years and serum testing has become an alternative to intradermal testing for many equine practitioners. However, tests vary in their sensitivity and specificity so that careful selection of an appropriate test is important.

✓ Testing for individual allergens rather than allergen groups is prudent to avoid immunotherapy with inappropriate allergens. It is impossible to tell which of the allergens in a particular reacting group are involved in the disease process.

✓ Results need to be interpreted in light of the clinical history of a patient. A horse with positive reactions to grass pollens only and a clinical history of nonseasonal pruritus for years in a temperate environment such as in England or Canada will most likely not benefit from allergen-specific immunotherapy.

✓ Intradermal testing is still widely considered the first choice for the identification of offending allergens in equine atopic dermatitis. Reliable serum tests have only recently been evaluated for the horse and our experience with these tests is still limited. Typically, more individual allergens are used in intradermal testing compared with in serum testing. The skin is the affected organ and thus it seems to be logical to test the organ affected. Finally, the input of a veterinary dermatologist in regards to the interpretation of test results and management of horses on allergen-specific immunotherapy is invaluable for many practitioners.

Diagnostic Trials

Diagnostic trials are very useful in veterinary dermatology. They are performed when a certain problem is suspected and the trial is either the only or the best way to diagnose the possible underlying disease. A response to the trial provides diagnostic evidence for or against the diagnosis. In some cases the importance of the change or restriction will not be apparent until relapse after discontinuation of the trial with subsequent resolution on restarting the trial (such as in diet trials). If there is no response to a well-conducted diagnostic trial, the suspected disease is unlikely. However, this can be frustrating to the owner and client education about the trial is key to success of this important technique.

Diet Trial

Indication

A diet trial is used to evaluate possible food adverse reaction. Food adverse reaction can occur to any food ingredient fed over a period of time. However, they are considered a rare problem in horses. Any horse with nonseasonal pruritus (particularly if the face or the neck are affected) or recurrent pyoderma could possibly have an underlying adverse food reaction.

Procedure

A diet trial for horses ideally consists of foods not previously fed! If this is not possible due to regular exposure of the horse to a number of different hay types, then alternatively one source such as Lucerne chaff, oat hay or grain should be fed exclusively for the first 3-4 weeks. If there is no response, a different source is fed for a further 3-4 weeks.

✓ The chosen hay needs to be fed exclusively! This will be the most difficult step as many horses are fed a huge number of different supplements. Concurrent supplements, vitamins and grains must be discontinued.

✓ It may take 3-4 weeks before response becomes evident.

☛ After initial improvement, a rechallenge with the previously fed diet is requisite to demonstrate that the food was the problem instead of incidental factors such as seasonal or environmental changes, or concurrent medication. If clinical signs recur within 2 weeks and resolve again after reinstitution of the diet trial, a diagnosis of food reaction is confirmed.

Insect-Control Trial

Indication

An aggressive insect-control trial should be completed in any horse with suspected insect-bite hypersensitivities. *Culicoides* flies are the most common cause of insect bite hypersensitivity, although hypersensitivities to other insects such as mosquitoes or black flies are possible. Any horse with pruritus, urticaria, and/or a papular or crusty dermatitis should undergo an insect control trial.

Procedure

✔ The horse needs to be treated regularly with an insecticide. This may require an increase in the frequency of administration above the manufacturer's recommendations. Insect repellants such as benzoyl benzoate or permethrin applied to blankets or body may provide some extra benefit. Which products are most suited, depends on the individual circumstances. More details are provided on p.78.

✔ As *Culicoides* spp. are most active at dusk and dawn, stabling the horse during these hours will be important, stables should be screened with fine mesh.

🖐 *Culicoides* spp. can pass through regular mesh, therefore a very fine mesh must be used.

✔ Rugs or blankets may offer some protection.

✔ *Culicoides* spp. do not fly well against air currents, so a fan located in the doorway and directed away from the stable can be helpful.

✔ Relocating the horse to a windy paddock away from standing water may help.

✔ At the start of the trial, I often prescribe 5 to 7 days of prednisolone at 1 mg/kg bodyweight daily to hasten clinical response.

✔ If there is good response to the trial, insect-bite hypersensitivity is present and the insect control may be tapered to the minimum required.

✔ Remember that the required minimum treatment typically varies seasonally in temperate climates, as does the insect load.

✔ Response should be apparent after 3-4 weeks of the trial, in many horses with insect bite hypersensitivity relief is noted after a few days already.

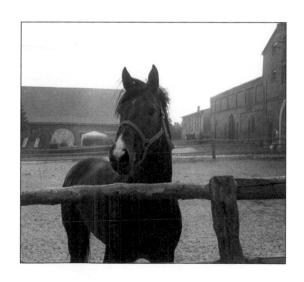

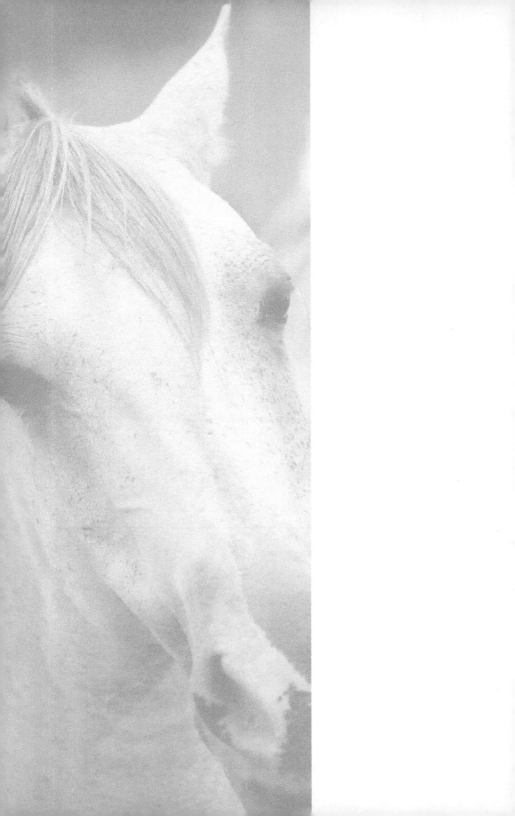

Section 2

The Approach to Common Dermatologic Presentations

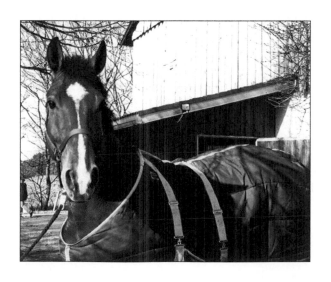

In this section, I present an approach to various common clinical presentations in equine dermatology. I begin each chapter in this section with general comments, followed by tables containing common differential diagnoses, their clinical features, diagnostic procedures of choice, treatment, and prognosis. I have attempted to list diseases in order of prevalence. Diseases marked with an asterisk are potentially difficult to diagnose or manage and may require referral to a veterinary dermatologist or equine specialist center.

This is not a textbook of equine dermatology, and thus the tables do not contain extensive detail but rather a concise overview of the important features of the more common diseases. The flow charts at the end of the chapters are concise and simplified to facilitate the use of this book by the equine practitioner in the field. They will be useful in most patients, but remember that some horses may not read the textbooks or follow the rules. It is the purpose of this book to guide you in diagnosis and formulation of a treatment plan, but your clinical acumen, examination, and communication skills remain the most crucial instruments for success in your daily practice.

The Pruritic Horse

Key Questions

Changes in behavior such as rubbing, kicking and biting are all indicative of pruritus. On physical examination, hair loss and/or excoriations are the most common clinical sequelae of itching.

All questions discussed in the first section may be relevant for a pruritic horse.

Many equine skin dermatoses are pruritic. The most common cause of pruritus in the horse is ectoparasite hypersensitivity. Hypersensitivities to environmental allergens and occasionally food components also occur. And finally horses with bacterial or fungal infections or occasionally with immune-mediated skin disease may also be pruritic. A thorough work-up will lead to diagnosis, prognosis and therapy based on the cause and an approach preferable to symptomatic treatment. Table 2-1 presents skin diseases in which pruritus is a prominent feature.

Table 2-1

Differential Diagnoses, Commonly Affected Sites, Diagnostic Tests, Treatment Options, and Prognoses for the Pruritic Horse

DISEASE	COMMONLY AFFECTED SITES	DIAGNOSTIC TESTS	TREATMENT	PROGNOSIS
Insect hypersensitivity (one of the most common skin disorders in the horse. *Culicoides* or *Simulium* spp. are the most common causative insects)	Pruritus and crusted papules on the ventrum or head/mane/tail/dorsum (depending on species), pruritus worst at dusk and dawn, self trauma leads to alopecia and excoriations (Figure 2-1)	History, physical examination, ectoparasite treatment trial	Insect repellants, screened stabling, protective blanketing and head gear, glucocorticoids (see p. 78).	From good to guarded, depending completely on the severity of the disease, length of the insect season and most importantly owner's ability to prevent exposure
Atopic dermatitis (hypersensitivity to airborne allergens)	Urticaria and/or pruritus (Figures 2-2, 2-3, and 2-4)	Diagnosis based on history, physical examination, and ruling out other pruritic dermatoses. Intradermal test or serum quantification of allergen-specific IgE identify offending allergens and allow formulation of immunotherapy	Allergen-specific immunotherapy, antihistamines, essential fatty acids, glucocorticoids (see pp. 74-78).	Poor for cure, good to guarded for management, depending on the horse and owner
Pediculosis (caused by biting lice [*Damalina equi*] or sucking lice [*Haematopinus asini*])	Dorsum, neck, tail, limbs (Figures 2-5, 2-6, and 2-7)	Microscopic evaluation of groomings	Fipronil or pyrethroid sprays, ivermectin beyond the life cycle (thus for at least 4 weeks), organophosphate rinses. All contact horses need to be treated (see p.79).	Good
Drug reaction	Urticaria, papules and/or pruritus, may start at mucocutaneous junctions	Usually presumptive through avoidance, biopsy may be helpful.	Discontinue and avoid drug, glucocorticoids may be beneficial.	Good
Trombiculidiasis (fairly common, only larvae of chiggers (harvest mites, *Trombicula affreddugesi* or *Neotrombicula autumnalis*) are parasitic, adults infest vegetation only.)	Papules, wheals and pruritus on head and legs, in temperate climates in summer to autumn	Microscopic evaluation of groomings, visualization of orange larvae (which only spend a short period on the host)	Prevention of reinfestation, insecticides and glucocorticoids concurrently for active infestation to treat the larvae and the inflammation associated with the infestation.	Good, but problem may be recurrent

41

Table 2-1 Continued

Disease	Commonly Affected Sites	Diagnostic Tests	Treatment	Prognosis
Chorioptes equi (common leg and tail mange)	Occurs more frequently in winter with scaling, alopecia and pruritus on distal legs, ventral abdomen (Figure 2-8)	Superficial skin scrapings (may be difficult to find)	Ivermectin helpful, but not curative. Fipronil spray, lime sulfur 2% rinses, organophosphate rinses (see p. 79). All contact horses need to be treated.	Good
Psoroptes equi (Body mange)	Seborrhea and/or pruritus with papules, alopecia, crusts and excoriation of the mane, body and tail	Superficial skin scrapings	Ivermectin, pyrethrin, pyrethroids, organophosphate or lime sulfur rinses (see p. 79). All contact horses need to be treated.	Good
Psoroptes hippotis (Ear mange)	Otitis externa and head shaking	Microscopic evaluation of ear wax	Ivermectin (see p. 79).	Good
Dermanyssus gallinae (uncommon disease caused by poultry mites living in the environment)	Papules, pruritus and crusts on legs, face and ventrum in horses with contact to poultry, poultry sheds or yards	Microscopic evaluation of groomings, superficial skin scrapings	Insecticides, but reinfestation needs to be prevented by eliminating the poultry sheds or environmental treatment.	Good
Onchocerciasis (used to be common prior to routine ivermectin use, caused by microfilaria of *Onchocerca cervicalis* transmitted by biting insects)	Alopecia, scaling, crusting, plaques, erosions or ulcers on ventral midline, face, neck, withers (Figure 2-9)	History, examination, response to therapy, biopsy, poor deworming	Fenbendazole, mebendazole, ivermectin	Good
Food adverse reaction (rarely diagnosed, as adequate elimination diets are rarely performed in horses)	General or perianal pruritus, urticaria (Figure 2-10)	Food elimination trials	Avoidance of allergens	Good
Generalized granulomatous disease or sarcoidosis (exfoliative dermatitis and wasting with systemic granulomatous inflammation of unknown etiology)	Pruritic exudative coronitis and dermatitis with alopecia and hyperkeratosis, weight loss, depression, pyrexia (Figure 2-11)	Low albumin and high plasma fibrinogen, biopsy	Glucocorticoids (see p. 74).	Spontaneous remission and response to glucocorticoids reported as well as nonresponsive disease

Figure 2-1 Papules and crusts on the neck of a 12 year old female Mule with insect bite hypersensitivity.

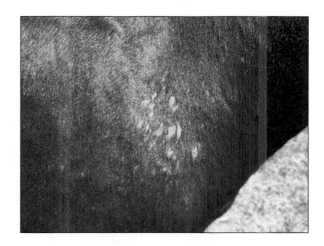

Figure 2-2 Trunkal urticaria of a horse.

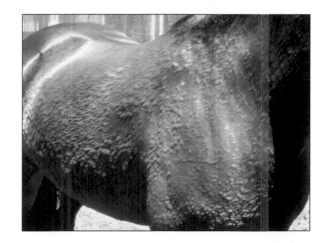

Figure 2-3 Urticarial hives on the lateral chest.

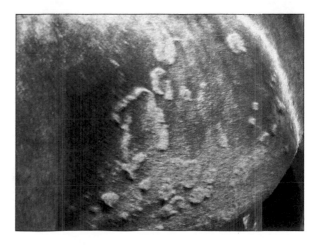

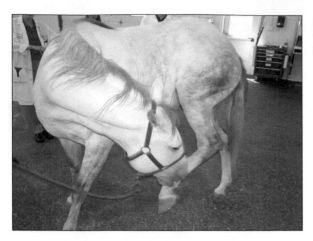

Figure 2-4 Pruritus with "nibbling" of distal limbs in an 11 year old mare.

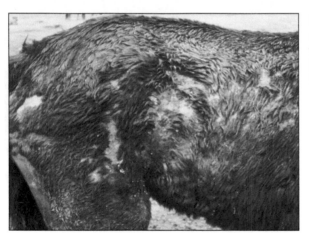

Figure 2-5 Multifocal alopecia due to self trauma in a horse with lice. (Courtesy of Dr. John Cheney.)

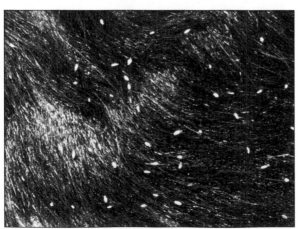

Figure 2-6 Close up of a lice infested horse. Note the numerous lice eggs or nits. (Courtesy of Dr. John Cheney.)

Figure 2-7 Excoriation and focal alopecia due to lice infestation. (Courtesy of Dr. Josie Traub-Dargatz.)

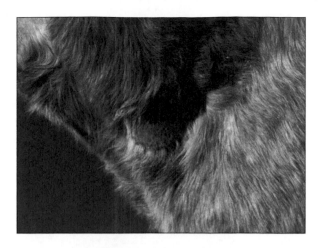

Figure 2-8 Erythema and alopecia associated with *Chorioptes equi* in a Percheron mare. (Courtesy of Dr. Rod Rosychuk.)

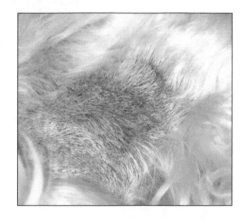

Figure 2-9 Alopecia, crusting, and focal ulceration on the face of a horse with oncocerciasis. (Courtesy of Dr. Josie Traub-Dargatz.)

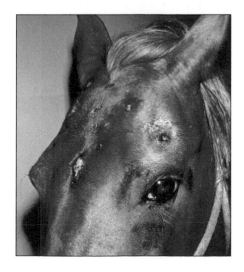

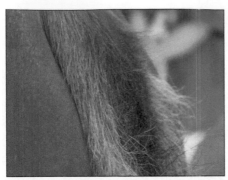

Figure 2-10 Tail rubbing and hypotrichosis due to allergic pruritus.

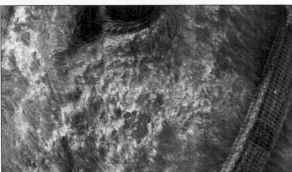

Figure 2-11 Alopecia and crusting due to generalized granulomatous disease in a 5 year old Thoroughbred. (Courtesy of Dr. Ann Hargis.)

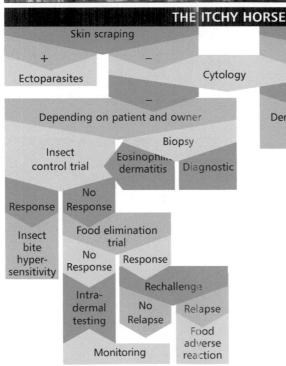

The Itchy Horse.

The Horse with Papules, Scales, or Crusts

Key Questions

✓ *How old was the patient when clinical signs were first recognized?*

✓ *How long has the disease been present and how did it progress?*

✓ *Is the horse pruritic?*

✓ *Is the disease seasonal?*

✓ *Are there other clinical signs such as sneezing or coughing?*

✓ *Do other horses have regular contact with this horse or share tack or grooming equipment? Do they have any skin disease or pruritus?*

✓ *Is there any correlation of clinical signs to humidity and/or rainfall?*

✓ *Was the disease treated before? If so, which drugs were used and how successful was the treatment?*

✓ *Does the horse get better with a change in environment (other paddock, stabling, etc.)*

Papules are uncommon, pustules rare, but both lesions typically develop into crusts. However, some diseases are characterized by papules that do not typically develop further into crusts (such as erythema multiforme), other diseases typically show crusting as their predominant symptom (pemphigus foliaceus), or are characterized by scaling and crusting. Table 2-2 lists the major differential diagnoses for a horse with papules, scales, or crusts.

Many diseases are associated with scaling. Primary seborrhea in the horse is rare and occurs as mane and tail seborrhea or generalized.

Crusting develops as a consequence of serum exudation and/or exocytosis of inflammatory cells. Examples would be infectious diseases such as dermatophytosis or immune-mediated diseases such as pemphigus foliaceus. These diseases may be pruritic; see the approach to the pruritic horse on page 40. Skin scrapings and cytology are always indicated to rule out evidence for infections, ectoparasites or possibly pemphigus foliaceus.

Table 2-2
Differential Diagnoses, Commonly Affected Sites, Recommended Diagnostic Tests, Treatment Options and Prognosis in a Horse with Papules, Scales, or Crusts

DISEASE	COMMONLY AFFECTED SITES	DIAGNOSTIC TESTS	TREATMENT	PROGNOSIS
Dermatophilosis (common, caused by *Dermatophilus congolensis* in association with moist conditions and/or trauma)	Alopecia, pustules and characteristic paint brush-like crusting either ventrally or dorsally (depending on the feeding habits of the species locally or (less commonly) on the hind cannon regions (muddy paddocks) (Figure 2-12, 2-13 and 2-14)	Cytology, culture (can be difficult, see page 21), culture, biopsy	Topical antiseptics/ antimicrobials, systemic antibiotics, keep horse dry (see pp. 70-73).	Fair
Dermatophytosis (common and frequently caused by *Trichophyton equinum*)	Expanding alopecia or papules with scaling and crusting on the face, neck, dorsal trunk and girth area (Figures 2-15, 2-16 and 2-17)	Trichogram, fungal culture	Antifungal shampoos and rinses to minimize contagious potential and environmental contamination (see p. 70).	Good
Bacterial folliculitis (caused by coagulase-positive staphylococci, typically secondary to trauma or less commonly underlying disease and most common in spring and summer)	Painful papules, pustules, crusts and/or ulcers in the saddle and/or tack area (Figures 2-18 and 2-19)	Cytology, culture, in selected cases biopsy	Clipping and cleaning, topical antibacterial agents, systemic antibiotics (see pp. 70-73).	Good, may be recurrent problem in some horses
Mane and tail seborrhea (an uncommon primary keratinization defect)	Moderate to severe scaling and crusting of rump, neck and head	Clinical presentation and biopsy	Topical antiseborrheic shampoos	Good for clinical management, poor for cure
Pemphigus foliaceus (uncommon autoimmune disorder affecting keratinocyte adhesion)	Annular erosions with scales and crusts, initially affecting face, neck and limbs, then generalizing. Edema of distal limbs and ventrum (Figures 2-20, 2-21, 2-22, 2-23 and 2-24).	Biopsy	Immunosuppressive therapy (see p. 80).	Good to guarded in foals (many may stay in remission after cessation of therapy), guarded to poor in older horses
Equine coital exanthema (contagious venereal skin disease caused by equine herpes virus)	Papules, pustules and crusts on prepuce, vulva, nose and/or mouth (Figure 2-25)	Serum neutralization, complement fixation, virus isolation	Iodine solution topically. Do not breed the horse until lesions completely resolved	Poor for cure, recurrences occur in stressful situations

Disease	Clinical signs	Diagnosis	Treatment	Prognosis
Chorioptes equi (common leg and tail mange)	frequently occurs in winter with scaling, alopecia and pruritus on distal limbs, abdomen,	Superficial skin scrapings	Ivermectin helpful, but not curative. Fipronil spray, lime sulfur 2% rinses, organophosphate rinses (see p. 79).	Good
Onchocerciasis (rare since introduction of ivermectin, caused by microfilaria of Onchocerca cervicalis transmitted by biting insects)	Alopecia, pruritus, scaling, crusting, plaques, erosions and/or ulcers on ventral midline, face, neck, withers (see Figure 2-9)	History, examination, response to therapy, biopsy, poor deworming	Ivermectin, fenbendazole, mebendazole, against microfilaria, short course of glucocorticoids against exacerbation of signs due to destruction of microfilaria (see p. 79).	Good
Psoroptes equi (Body mange)	Seborrhea and/or pruritus with papules, alopecia, crusts and excoriation of the mane, body and tail	Superficial skin scrapings	Ivermectin, pyrethrin, pyrethroids, organophosphate or lime sulfur rinses (see p. 79).	Good
Verminous dermatitis (uncommon and caused by Pelodera strongyloides & Strongyloides westeri in young horses in poor hygienic conditions	Sudden onset of pruritus with papules, crusts and ulcers of legs	Deep skin scrapings, biopsy	Improved hygiene, topical glucocorticoids and antibiotics, deworming	Excellent
Generalized seborrhea (rare primary keratinization defect)	Moderate to severe scaling and crusting of rump, neck and head	Clinical presentation and biopsy	Topical antiseborrheic shampoos (see p.71).	Good for clinical management, poor for cure
Linear alopecia and keratosis (rare and possibly hereditary skin disease of unknown etiology)	Unilateral, linear, vertically oriented bands of alopecia and hyperkeratosis over the neck, shoulders and lateral thorax, lesions may be painful (Figure 2-26)	Clinical presentation and biopsy	Topical antiseborrheic treatment	Excellent for well-being, poor for cure
Generalized granulomatous disease or sarcoidosis (exfoliative dermatitis and wasting with systemic granulomatous inflammation of unknown etiology)	Pruritic exudative coronitis and dermatitis with alopecia and hyperkeratosis, weight loss, depression, pyrexia	Low albumin and high plasma fibrinogen, biopsy	Glucocorticoids (see p.74).	Spontaneous remission and response to glucocorticoids reported as well as nonresponsive disease
Equine viral papular disease (caused by an unspecified poxvirus reported only in North America and Australia)	Papules and crusts over trunk and scrotal skin	Biopsy, virus isolation from papules	None, spontaneous remission	Excellent

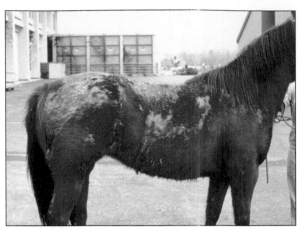

Figure 2-12
Dermatophilosis with dorsal alopecia and crusting. (Courtesy of Dr. Anthony Stannard.)

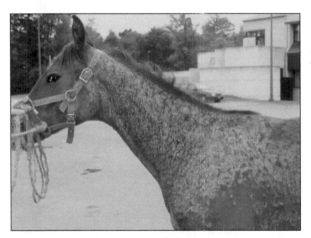

Figure 2-13
Dermatophilosis with alopecia and crusting of the neck and shoulders. (Courtesy of Dr. Luc Beco)

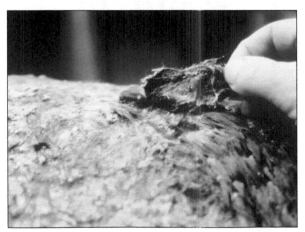

Figure 2-14
Crusts are easily lifted off the skin with equine dermatophilosis. (Courtesy of Dr. Hélène Amory.)

Figure 2-15
Focal crusting on the neck of a horse with dermatophytosis. (Courtesy of Dr. Sonya Bettenay.)

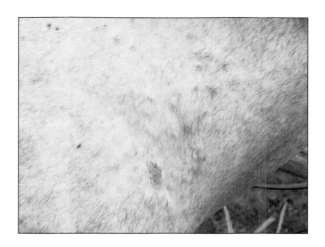

Figure 2-16 Alopecia, crusting, and ulceration on the face of a 4 year old Quarterhorse mare.

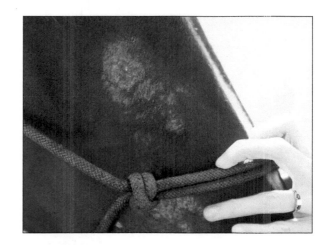

Figure 2-17 Close-up of the lesion in Figure 2-16.

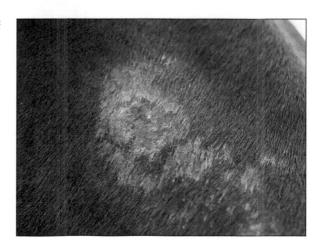

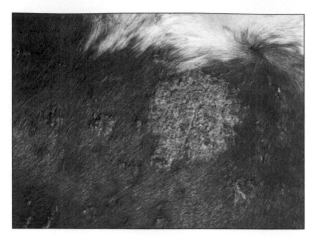

Figure 2-18 Crusting and alopecia due to bacterial pyoderma in a 2 year old American Paint mare.

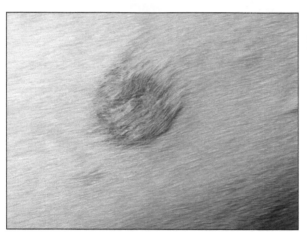

Figure 2-19 A crusted plaque on the trunk of the mare in Figure 2-15.

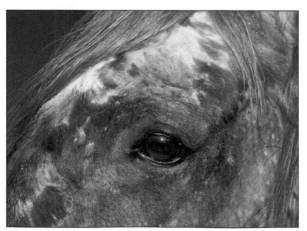

Figure 2-20 Alopecia and scaling on the face of an 8 year old Peruvian Paso gelding with pemphigus foliaceus.

Figure 2-21
The affected neck of the horse in Figure 2-20.

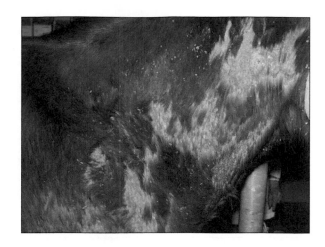

Figure 2-22 A 6 month old American Paint colt with pemphigus foliaceus.

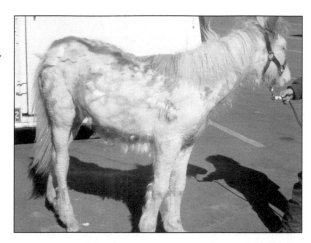

Figure 2-23 Close-up of Figure 2-22 showing alopecia, crusting, and focal erosions.

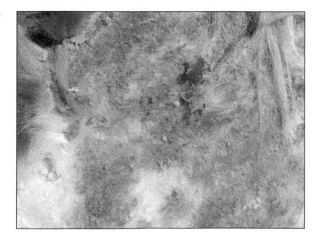

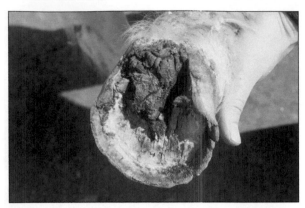

Figure 2-24
Contracted heel, proliferative frog, crusty coronary band, and overgrown hoof in the horse from Figure 2-22.

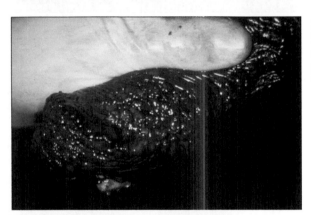

Figure 2-25 Papules on the penis of a horse with coital exanthema. (Courtesy of Dr. Josie Traub-Dargatz.)

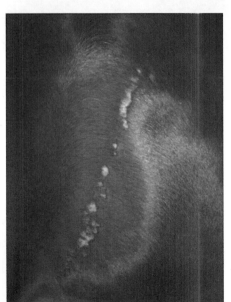

Figure 2-26 Equine linear alopecia and keratosis on the lateral chest. (Courtesy of Dr. Andrea Cannon.)

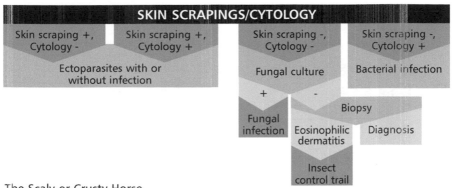

Skin scraping +, Cytology -	Skin scraping +, Cytology +	Skin scraping -, Cytology -	Skin scraping -, Cytology +
Ectoparasites with or without infection		Fungal culture	Bacterial infection

Fungal culture + → Fungal infection

Fungal culture - → Biopsy: Eosinophilic dermatitis / Diagnosis

Insect control trail

The Scaly or Crusty Horse.

The Horse with Nodules

Key Questions

✔ *How old was this horse when nodules were first recognized?*

✔ *How many nodules are there?*

✔ *How long have the nodules been present and how did they progress?*

✔ *Are there any other animals in contact with the affected horse?*

✔ *Were the nodules treated before? If so, which drugs were used and how successful was treatment?*

Differential Diagnoses

The differential diagnoses will be determined by the following: (1) Is there only one nodule (which increases the likelihood of neoplasia or infectious organisms gaining entry via wounds, such as mycetomas or pseudomycetomas) or are there multiple lesions (which may be due to sterile inflammatory diseases, more aggressive neoplastic disease or severe infection)? (2) Are draining tracts absent or present (increasing the likelihood of foreign bodies, severe bacterial or fungal infection, or sterile inflammatory disease)?

The approach to the horse with nodules is straightforward. History and clinical examination are followed by microscopic evaluation of impression smears (if draining tracts are present) and aspirates (in any horse with nodules). In some patients, cytology will reveal an infectious organism or classic neoplastic cells and thus a diagnosis. In most patients, cytologic examination will narrow the list of differential diagnoses, but a biopsy will be necessary to reach a definitive diagnosis. With nodular lesions, a complete excision of one or several nodules is ideal where possible. If draining tracts are present and/or cytology indicates possible infection, a culture and sensitivity may be useful as well. Deep tissue should be submitted rather than a culture swab.

Table 2-3

Differential Diagnoses, Commonly Affected Sites, Recommended Diagnostic Tests, Treatment Options and Prognosis in a Horse with Nodules

Disease	Commonly Affected Sites	Diagnostic Tests	Treatment	Prognosis
Abscess (common, often due to trauma, and caused by *Corynebacterium pseudotuberculosis* or *Clostridium equi* or systemic infection for example with *Streptococcus equi*)	One or multiple nodules (Figure 2-27)	Aspiration cytology	Hot compresses, surgical drainage, antibiotics after drainage or in very early stages	Depends on organism involved and severity of infection
Eosinophilic granuloma (most common nonneoplastic nodular equine skin disease, local reaction to insect bites may be the cause in some horses)	Single or multiple, subcutaneous firm nodules (Figures 2-28 & 2-29)	Biopsy	Surgical excision, intralesional or systemic glucocorticoids	Good
Hypodermiasis (common ectoparasitic disease in horses and cattle in some parts of the world due to larvae of *Hypoderma* spp.)	Initially firm subcutaneous nodules over the withers of younger horses, later softening with development of a breathing pore	Examination, consistent history (affected cattle in same area)	Ivermectin prevents larval migration and development, surgical excision	Excellent, but anaphylaxis is possible after drug-induced parasite death
Parafilariasis (common disease in many countries caused by the nematode *Parafilaria multipapulosa*)	Papules and nodules occur in spring and summer over the neck and rump, discharge a bloody exudate and then heal	Direct smears, biopsy	Ivermectin	Excellent
Habronemiasis (common and due to cutaneous penetration of Habronema larvae)	Seasonal spring/summer occurrence of ulcerating cutaneous nodules and ulcers periocularly, on the penis/prepuce and in areas of trauma	History, examination, cytology, biopsy	Glucocorticoids, ivermectin, surgical resection	Good

Condition	Clinical presentation	Diagnosis	Treatment	Prognosis
Squamous cell carcinoma (a common skin tumor arising from keratinocytes in sun-damaged skin)	Solitary nonhealing ulcers or proliferative masses in lightly pigmented and sparsely haired skin (Figures 2-30 & 2-31).	Cytology, biopsy	Surgical excision, cryosurgery (best with lesions <2cm), 5-fluorouracil (5% cream), laser surgery	Fair to good, if lesions are small and excision is possible, guarded to poor with large lesions
Sarcoid (most common equine skin tumor, locally aggressive, viral (BPV 1,2) fibroblastic cell origin)	Nodular, proud flesh-like, wart-like or alopecic and scaly lesions are all possible and most commonly seen on head, neck, limbs and ventrum. (Figures 2-32 & 2-33).	Biopsy (although biopsy may stimulate growth of remaining tissue and transform quiescent tissue into proliferative lesions)	Surgical excision, cryosurgery, laser therapy, bleomycin, cisplatin, imiquimod, mycobacterial products	Good, if treatment does not lead to aggressive behavior, otherwise guarded to poor
Melanoma (a common malignant tumor seen most frequently in older gray horses)	Nodules, plaques or verrucous lesions most commonly seen under the tail and in the perianal region, but also on the head and distal limbs (Figures 2-34 & 2-35).	Clinical presentation, cytology, biopsy	Surgical excision for solitary melanomas, in multiple melanomas cryosurgery or cimetidine may be useful	Poor for cure, if not completely excised solitary lesion. Slow progression in many horses.
Ulcerative lymphangitis (infrequent bacterial infection of cutaneous lymphatics)	Nodules on the distal limbs following lymphatic chains (most commonly hind limbs), which ulcerate and drain (Figure 2-36)	Clinical features, biopsy, culture	Exercise, surgical drainage and long term antibiotics	Fair to guarded with early lesions, guarded to poor once significant fibrosis present
Bacterial granuloma (Pseudomycetoma, due to trauma and infection with Staphylococci)	Nodule with ulcerated surface and purulent discharge from sinuses, possibly development of exuberant granulation tissue	History, culture, biopsy	Surgical excision followed by antibiotic treatment	Good if complete surgical excision possible
Phaeohyphomycosis (rare and due to wound infection with Drechslera spicifera)	Small dark plaques and nodules, that may ulcerate and drain	Biopsy, fungal culture	Antifungal treatment with systemic iodides, with solitary lesions surgical excision is recommended	Poor
Mycetoma (rare and caused by fungal contamination of wounds by saprophytes such as Curvularia geniculata or Pseudoallescheria boydii)	Ulcerated nodules of ventrum, legs and head	Biopsy, culture	Surgical excision followed by oral potassium iodide	Guarded to poor
Sporotrichosis (an uncommon chronic infection of skin and lymphatics by Sporothrix schenkii)	Corded ulcerated subcutaneous nodules of lower legs	Cytology, culture, clinical presentation	Iodides	Good (if not disseminated) to guarded

continued

Table 2-3 continued

DISEASE	COMMONLY AFFECTED SITES	DIAGNOSTIC TESTS	TREATMENT	PROGNOSIS
Pythiosis (caused by *Pythium insidiosum*, an aquatic organism living in standing water in tropical environment and invading damaged tissue)	Pruritic dense granulation tissue with necrotic center, serosanginous discharge, and lymphangitis affecting the legs and ventrum	Biopsy, culture, PCR	Repeat surgical excision with concurrent iodide therapy	Poor
Amyloidosis (Rare primary deposition of amyloid in skin or upper respiratory tract, or secondary due to chronic immune stimulation typically leading to systemic amyloidosis without cutaneous involvement)	Nodules and plaques in skin and mucous membranes of upper respiratory tract, epistaxis (Figures 2-37 & 2-38)	Biopsy	None	Good for life (if only skin is affected), poor for remission

Figure 2-27
Corynebacterium equi abscess after an intramuscular injection in the pectoral area of a horse. (Courtesy of Dr. Josie Traub-Dargatz.)

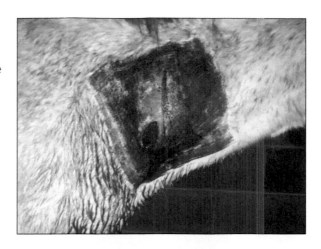

Figure 2-28 Eosinophilic granuloma on the chest. (Courtesy of Dr. Josie Traub-Dargatz.)

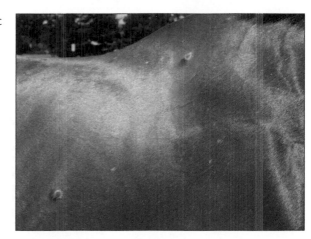

Figure 2-29 Close-up of eosinophlic granulomas. (Courtesy of Dr. Josie Traub-Dargatz.)

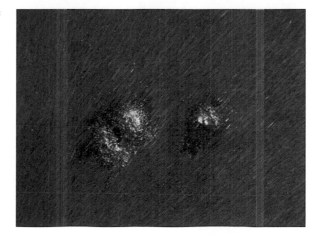

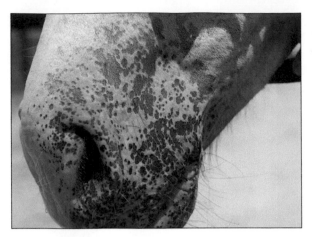

Figure 2-30 Actinic keratosis on the muzzle of an Appaloosa gelding.

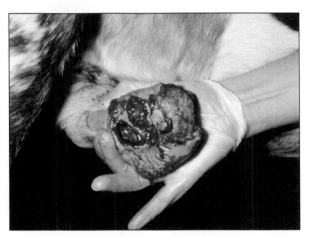

Figure 2-31 Squamous cell carcinoma on the penis of a horse. (Courtesy of Dr. Josie Traub-Dargatz.)

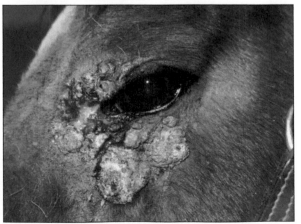

Figure 2-32 Nodules, crusts, and ulceration in the periocular area due to a sarcoid. (Courtesy of Dr. Josie Traub-Dargatz.)

Figure 2-33 Verrucous sarcoid. (Courtesy of Dr. Josie Traub-Dargatz.)

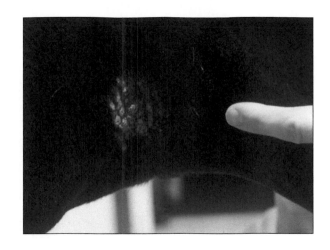

Figure 2-34 Large melanoma of the tail, perianal and perineal area in a grey mare.

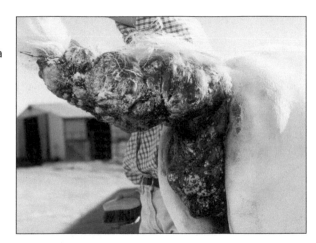

Figure 2-35 Melanoma on the muzzle of a horse. (Courtesy of Dr. Josie Traub-Dargatz.)

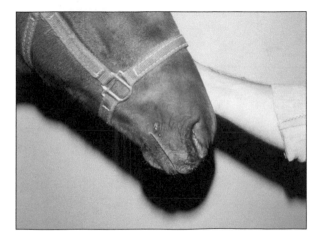

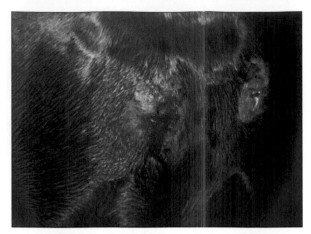

Figure 2-36 Ulcerative lymphangitis in a horse. (Courtesy of Dr. Andrea Cannon.)

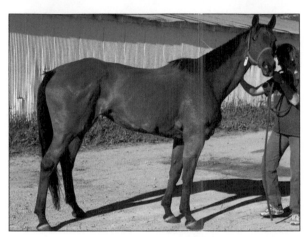

Figure 2-37 Amyloidosis in a 20 year old Thoroughbred mare.

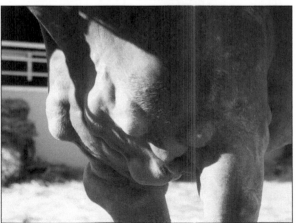

Figure 2-38 Close-up of the cranial chest of the mare in Figure 2-37.

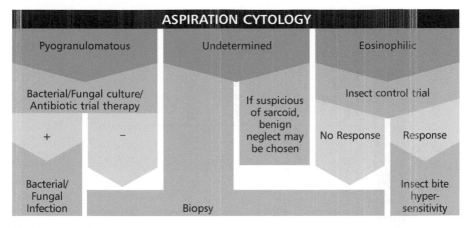

ASPIRATION CYTOLOGY		
Pyogranulomatous	Undetermined	Eosinophilic
Bacterial/Fungal culture/ Antibiotic trial therapy	If suspicious of sarcoid, benign neglect may be chosen	Insect control trial
+ —	No Response	Response
Bacterial/ Fungal Infection	Biopsy	Insect bite hyper- sensitivity

The Horse with Nodules.

The Horse with Alopecia

Many diseases are associated with alopecia in conjunction with pruritus and other lesions. This chapter discusses the approach to horses with clinically noninflammatory alopecias.

Key Questions

✓ *What breed is the horse?*

✓ *How old was this patient when clinical signs were first recognized?*

✓ *How long has the disease been present and how did it progress?*

✓ *On which part of the body did the problem start?*

✓ *Is the horse itchy?*

✓ *Is the disease seasonal?*

✓ *Was the disease treated before? If so, which drugs were used and how successful was treatment?*

If the alopecic horse is pruritic, but lacks other lesions, the approach is described on p.40 and is different from that used in an alopecic horse without pruritus. Many alopecias are characterized by dry skin and mild scaling which may or may not be pruritic. The use of moisturizers will help the dryness and may address concurrent pruritus. Differential diagnoses for noninflammatory and nonpruritic alopecias are outlined later in this section.

Table 2-4
Differential Diagnoses, Commonly Affected Sites, Recommended Diagnostic Tests, Treatment Options, and Prognosis in a Horse with Alopecia or Hypotrichosis

DISEASE	COMMONLY AFFECTED SITES	DIAGNOSTIC TESTS	TREATMENT	PROGNOSIS
Alopecia areata (uncommon cell-mediated response against hair matrix and follicular epithelium)	Focal, circular, partial or complete alopecia anywhere on the body or thinning of mane and/or tail (Figures 2-39, 2-40, and 2-41)	Biopsy	Topical steroids or tacrolimus may be of benefit	Fair to guarded for remission (spontaneous remission possible), excellent for well-being
Occult sarcoid (a common and locally aggressive, viral (BPV 1,2) fibroblastic tumor)	Roughly circular alopecia often with mild hyperkeratosis or small nodules (Figures 2-42 and 2-43)	Biopsy (although biopsy may trigger aggressive verrucous transformation)	Complete surgical excision, laser therapy, bleomycin, imiquimod, 5-fluorouracil	Unpredictable
Mane and tail dystrophy (probably genetic follicular dysplasia of mane and tail particularly common in Appaloosas)	Sparse thin hair coat of mane and tail	Biopsy	None	Excellent for well-being, poor for cure
Telogen defluxion (uncommon, stressfull event causes abrupt telogenization of follicles with subsequent hair loss 4-12 weeks later when telogen hairs are shed and new hairs grow in)	Symmetrical hypotrichosis or alopecia	History	None	Excellent

	Alopecia	History, trichogram	Removal of cause	Excellent, if cause can be removed
Anagen defluxion (uncommon, hairs break easily during anagen phase due to high fever, severe illness or antimitotic drugs)				
Demodicosis (rare and caused by a proliferation of Demodex caballi/equi due to immunosuppression associated with disease or long term glucocorticoid therapy	Asymptomatic patchy alopecia and scaling over the neck, shoulders and forelimbs	Deep skin scrapings, biopsy	Discontinue glucocorticoids, treat systemic disease, ivermectin	Depending on underlying disease

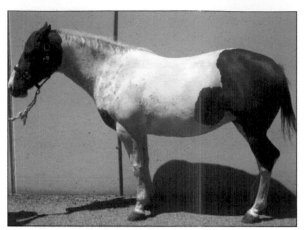

Figure 2-39 Alopecia areata causing multifocal alopecia on the trunk of a horse. (Courtesy of Dr. Josie Traub-Dargatz.)

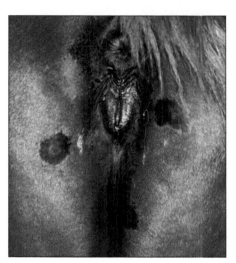

Figure 2-40 Alopecia in the perineal ara of a mare with alopecia areata. (Courtesy of Dr. Sonja Zabel.)

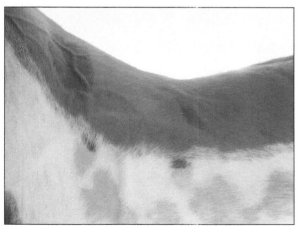

Figure 2-41 Multifocal alopecia on the neck and chest of a horse with alopecia areata. (Courtesy of Dr. Josie Traub-Dargatz.)

Figure 2-42 Flat sarcoid on the face of a 12 year old Quarterhorse. (Courtesy of Dr. Sonya Bettenay.)

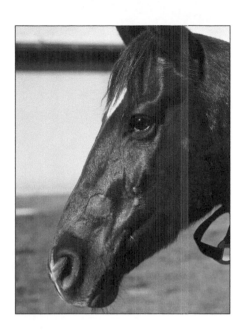

Figure 2-43 Close-up of the lesion in Figure 2-42. (Courtesy of Dr. Sonya Bettenay.)

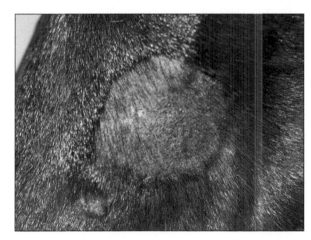

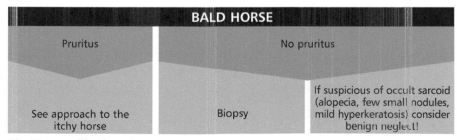

BALD HORSE		
Pruritus	No pruritus	
See approach to the itchy horse	Biopsy	If suspicious of occult sarcoid (alopecia, few small nodules, mild hyperkeratosis) consider benign neglect!

The Horse with Alopecia.

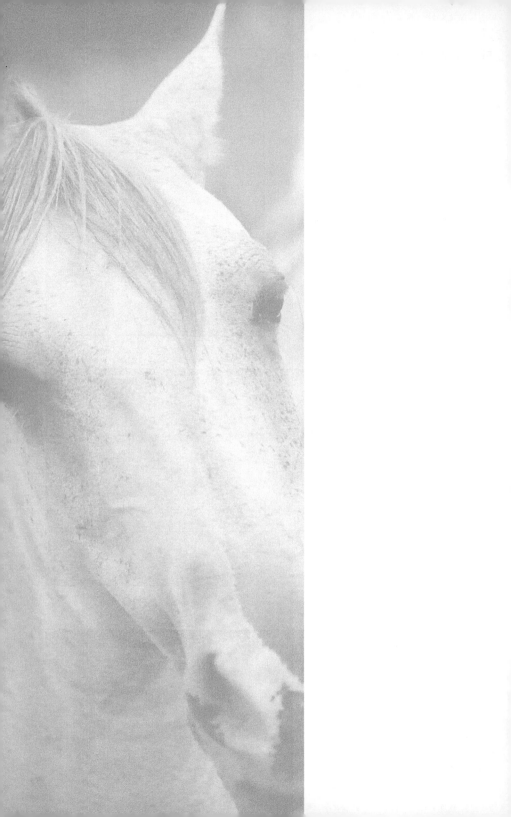

Section 3
Treatments

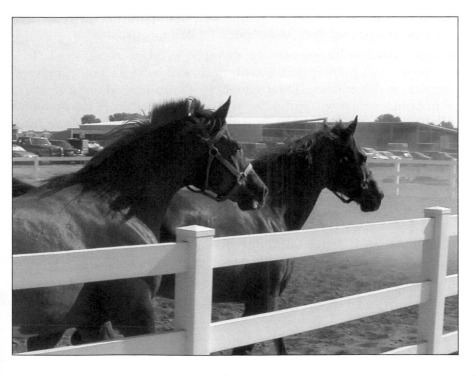

In this section, I will summarize the most common treatment modalities, their formulations (which may vary in different parts of the world), indications, and doses. Given that detailed discussion of individual drugs, their mechanisms of action, pharmacokinetics, and protocols is beyond the scope of this text, further reading may be required. Recommended Readings are listed in the back of the book.

Drugs marked with an asterisk are potentially dangerous and the clinician inexperienced with these medications may consider offering referral to a veterinary specialist or seeking further advice from a colleague with more knowledge about that particular agent.

Shampoo Therapy For Various Skin Conditions

Shampoo therapy can provide effective medical and cosmetic management of dermatoses. However, shampooing the whole body of a horse is a major undertaking and thus shampoo therapy is most commonly used for localized skin disease. Fungal and bacterial infections, allergies, as well as mane and tail seborrheas are the most common indication for shampoo therapy in equine practice. There are few adverse affects associated with shampoo therapy, although they are recognized. However, shampoo therapy is a symptomatic treatment, and rarely "cures" a dermatosis.

For best results, the appropriate shampoo needs to be selected. In addition, the veterinarian's instructions will have a significant impact on the efficacy. The frequency of bathing and duration of skin contact time will influence the obtained result. A minimum of 10-20 minutes of contact time is recommended. This is a long time for most horse owners. The shampoo may be applied thoroughly to affected areas and subsequently other tasks may be attended to for 10 minutes before rinsing the shampoo off completely for at least 5-10 minutes. The frequency of shampooing will vary with the severity and type of disease process. In general, the more severe the disease, the more frequently bathing is indicated.

The major reasons for failure of shampoo therapy are:

1. Lack of client compliance (frequency and/or duration of application)
2. Incorrect selection of shampoo for the disease process

Table 3-1
Selected Shampoo Types for the Treatment of Skin Disease in Equine Practice

SHAMPOO TYPE	COMMENTS	INDICATIONS	FREQUENCY OF ADMINISTRATION
Chlorhexidine	Antibacterial, not inactivated by organic matter, not irritating or drying.	Bacterial infections	q 1-14 days
Benzoyl peroxide	Degreasing (and thus drying), keratolytic. In horses with dry or normal skin, a moisturizer must be used after the shampoo! May be irritating, particularly in concentrations over 3%.	Bacterial infections, greasy seborrheic disorders	q 7-14 days
Iodine	Antifungal, antibacterial, virucidal, sporicidal, degreasing, but also staining and potentially irritating!	Superficial bacterial and fungal infections. May also be helpful in decreasing environmental contamination with fungi.	q 7-14 days
Sulfur	Keratoplastic and keratolytic, antibacterial and mildly antifungal. Synergistic with salicylic acid.	Seborrhea sicca, seborrheic dermatitis	q 3-14 days
Salicylic acid	Keratolytic, mildly anti-inflammatory, synergistic action with sulfur.	Seborrhea sicca, seborrheic dermatitis	q 3-14 days
Tar	Keratoplastic and keratolytic, antipruritic and degreasing. In horses with dry or normal skin, needs to be followed with a moisturizer.	Seborrheic dermatitis, seborrhea oleosa	q 3-14 days
Colloidal oatmeal	Hydrates the stratum corneum.	Pruritic skin disease, dry skin	q 2-14 days

Treatment of Bacterial Infections

✓ Trauma is a common cause of bacterial skin infection in horses. *Streptococcus equi* or *Corynebacterium pseudotuberculosis* are the most common organisms found in abscesses. Streptococci and staphylococci and are most commonly seen with folliculitis.

☞ Abscesses initially should not be treated with systemic antibiotics; poulticing and hot compresses will speed up the development of a mature abscess. Appropriate drainage is most important, after which antibacterial treatment may be beneficial.

☞ Dermatophilosis is a common surface bacterial infection caused by *Dermatophilus congolensis* and typically associated with prolonged moist conditions. Recurrences will be common if exposure to moisture is not reduced.

✓ Horses with chronic allergies or immune-mediated dermatoses may develop secondary bacterial folliculitis that exacerbates these conditions and necessitates antibacterial treatment.

✓ Hyperadrenocorticism is a common cause of oral abscessation.

✓ Not all available antibiotics are useful for skin infections so that spectrum of activity as well as pharmacology of the different antibacterial drugs have to be considered.

☞ Proper dosage and proper duration are important for the success of antibacterial therapy. Although many bacterial infections in the horse respond to short courses of antibiotics, longer courses may be needed in some patients, particularly with deep infections such as abscesses or bacterial granulomas.

✓ Pyodermas can, at least initially, be treated empirically. If appropriate therapy does not resolve the condition, a culture and sensitivity is indicated.

✓ Each sample for culture and sensitivity should be accompanied by cytologic examination and culture results interpreted in light of the cytology, as growth of different microorganisms does not indicate necessarily that they are present in significant numbers *in vivo*.

✓ Macrolids such as erythromycin and lincomycin may cause severe diarrhea due to their effects on bacterial flora in the large colon. Tetracyclines also should be used with caution.

✓ Enrofloxacine should not be used in foals due to possible cartilage erosions.

Table 3-2
Selected Antibiotics in Equine Dermatology

Drug	Formulation	Indications	Adverse Effects	Dose
Penicillin G	300,000 IU/ml for injection	Infections with most gram-positive and gram-negative cocci (not penicillinase producing strains), Clostridium sp., Fusobacterium and Actinomyces.	Hypersensitivity reactions	20,000-40,000 IU/kg (10 ml/70-150 kg bodyweight) IM q 12 h
Penicillin V	500-mg tablets	Infections with Actinomyces, most spirochetes and gram-positive and gram-negative cocci, which do not produce penicillinase.	Gastrointestinal signs with oral administration, hypersensitivity reactions	40-60 mg/kg (10 tablets/100kg body-weight) q 8 h
Trimethoprim/ sulfadiazine	800mg trimethoprim/ 160mg sulfadiazine, 48% sterile injection	Infections with gram-positive bacteria (streptococci, staphylococci). Many gram-negative organisms of the family Enterobacteriaceae are also susceptible (but not Pseudomonas aeruginosa).	Transient pruritus, diarrhea, hypersensitivities, blood dyscrasias	20-30 mg/kg (1 tablet/ 30-50 kg bodyweight) q 24 h; 15-20 mg/kg (10 ml/250-350 kg bodyweight) IV q 12-24 h
Chloramphenicol	1000mg tablets, 100 mg/ml as sodium succinate powder for injection	Infections with most gram-positive and gram-negative cocci, Clostridium sp., Fusobacterium and Nocardia.	Bone marrow toxicity	50 mg/kg q 8 h (10 tablets/200 kg bodyweight)
Cephalexin	1000-mg tablets	Infections with streptococci, staphylococci, Actinobacillus, Corynebacteria (except C. equi)	Vomiting and diarrhea; very rarely excitability, tachypnea or blood dyscrasias	20-30 mg/kg q 8 h
Enrofloxacine	136-mg tablets	Infections with staphylococci and many gram-negative bacteria	Cartilage erosions in growing foals	2.5-5 mg/kg q 24 h

Treatment of Pruritus

Glucocorticoids

Glucocorticoids are very commonly used in the treatment of skin conditions.

At anti-inflammatory dosages, they decrease inflammatory cell activity and migration.

Corticosteroids are effective in most, but not all horses with atopic disease and resolve the symptoms at least initially at reasonably low dosages. Insect allergic horses will often respond to these drugs. Prednisolone is preferable to prednisone as the latter is not efficacious in some horses.

Glucocorticoids can be considered in animals with mild seasonal pruritus of 1 to 2 months duration that is controlled with anti-inflammatory dosages (<0.2 mg/kg) of prednisolone every other day.

Every other day therapy is preferred over daily drug administration because it is thought to lower the chances of iatrogenic hyperadrenocorticism.

I use prednisolone at anti-inflammatory doses for severely affected horses in the short term to break the "itch-scratch cycle." However, the need to increase the dosage over time to control the clinical signs occurs in most of these patients. This, combined with the potential side effects, makes glucocorticoids a poor long-term choice for atopic horses. Adverse effects may include laminitis, in addition to increased susceptibility to infection, and other well-known symptoms of iatrogenic hyperadrenocorticism such as polydipsia, polyuria, or poor wound healing. Drugs should always be tapered to the lowest effective dose. Performance horses will have to be withdrawn for treatment prior to events (check withdrawal periods carefully!).

Table 3-3
Selected Glucocorticoids and Their Dosage

DRUG	FORMULATION	STARTING DOSE
Prednisolone	20-mg, 50-mg tablets, granules	0.2-1 mg/kg q 24-48 h orally
Methylprednisolone	100-mg tablets	0.2-1 mg/kg q 24-48 h orally
Dexamethasone	4-mg tablets	0.05-0.2 mg/kg q 48-72 h orally
Triamcinolone	8-mg tablets	0.01-0.05 mg/kg q 48-72 h orally

Antihistamines

Antihistamines are useful adjunctive agents in the management of pruritic horses with atopic dermatitis, urticaria, and possibly insect bite hypersensitivity. The classic antihistamines act by blocking H1-receptors. First-generation antihistamines also have an anticholinergic, sedative, and local anesthetic effects. Second-generation antihistamines penetrate less through the blood brain barrier or have a low affinity for the brain, compared with the action on peripheral H1-receptors. Thus, they are effective yet produce less sedation. Due to their cost, second-generation antihistamines are rarely used in horses.

The advantage of antihistamines is the rare occurrence of adverse effects. Drowsiness is the most common finding and may decrease after 2 to 3 days of therapy. Thus, it may be worthwhile to continue treatment for several days before final evaluation. Less common side effects include gastrointestinal signs. Due to the anticholinergic properties of terfenadine and cyproheptadine and possible induction of hypertension, these drugs should not be used in horses with severe cardiovascular disease. Hydroxyzine is teratogenic and must not be given to pregnant mares.

The necessity of frequent administration (two to three times daily) and the relatively high cost limit their long-term use in many horses. My antihistamine of choice in horses is hydroxyzine. However, its use in show horses is prohibited by some horse associations in the United States.

🖐 The potential success rate can be increased by trying several different antihistamines sequentially because horses may be responsive to one antihistamine but not to another.

✍ Because the withdrawal time of antihistamines before an intradermal test is much shorter than that of glucocorticoids, they can be used to relieve pruritus during the preparation time where the latter are contraindicated.

Table 3-4
Selected Antihistamines Used in the Treatment of Equine Hypersensitivities

DRUG	FORMULATION	COMMENTS	DOSE
Chlorpheniramine	4 mg tablets	Potentially sedating	40-100 mg/500 kg q 8-12 h
Diphenhydramine	25 mg tablets	Potentially sedating	500 mg/500 kg q 8-12 h
Hydroxyzine	50 mg capsules	Also inhibits mast cell degranulation, and is tricyclic antidepressant and teratogenic!!	400-800 mg/500 kg q 8-12 h
Amitriptylline	50 mg tablets		50 mg/500 kg q 12 h

Allergen-specific Immunotherapy*

Specific immunotherapy was introduced to veterinary medicine in the1960s. Based on several reports, a good to excellent response is seen in at least 60-70% of the horses.

In specific immunotherapy, an individual is exposed to extracts of antigens to which it has shown an allergic reaction. This exposure starts at low concentrations that are increased gradually over time, and after reaching a maintenance dose, are either continued indefinitely or slowly tapered.

Considerations Before Beginning Allergen-Specific Immunotherapy

Several key issues need to be discussed with the owners before they consider allergen-specific immunotherapy or "allergy shots".

The success rate: 20-30% of the patients will do extremely well and thrive with no additional therapy; 40-50% of the patients do well, even though occasional additional treatments such as antihistamines and/or glucocorticoids are needed. Owners are happy with the improvement achieved and consider the allergy shots worthwhile, although therapy may be lifelong.

The cost: This may vary depending on the country of practice, the horse's allergies, the extracts used, and the dose rates needed. In general, allergy shots are comparatively inexpensive for horses since the doses used are similar to those in dogs, while most other medications are administered depending on weight and so are much more expensive for horses than for small animals. Veterinary dermatologists are a good source of information for approximate expense.

The time to improvement: First improvement may be seen as early as 4 weeks into therapy and as late as 12 months after starting the allergy shots. On average, improvement is expected after 4 to 6 months.

The duration of treatment: Allergen-specific immunotherapy is a long term therapy! Although in some horses it may be discontinued after 2 years without recurrence of clinical signs, most horses receive injections long term.

The involvement: Atopic horses are "high maintenance" and as such need constant care, most likely at least initially regular rechecks and concurrent medication. Allergy shots are not an easy way out, but at this point may be the best of many available treatments, all of which involve long-term administration of medications of some sort.

Points to Remember if You Have Patients on Immunotherapy

Glucocorticoids may be given on an occasional basis at anti-inflammatory dosages without interfering with therapy. Antihistamines and antimicrobials do not interfere with immunotherapy, thus they may be, and often are, used concurrently.

✓ If there is a regular increase in pruritus after the injection, the dose and frequency may need to be adjusted. Decreased doses may be helpful.

✓ If there is a regular increase in pruritus before the injection is due, and reduction after the injection of allergen extract, the time interval between the injections is probably too long and should be shortened.

✓ If there is no response to allergen-specific immunotherapy after 6-9 months, I recommend that you contact your nearest veterinary dermatologist for advice while there is still sufficient vaccine left to change the dose and frequency of the injections by adjusting them to the needs of that particular patient. Many patients need an approach suiting their particular requirements and the help of a veterinarian experienced in immunotherapy may be of great benefit.

I believe that allergen-specific immunotherapy is the best available treatment for atopic dermatitis in the horse, but it will only be successful if owners and veterinarians have realistic expectations and are prepared to put in significant effort over a period that sometimes extends over many months. Only then will maximal benefit be achieved! In as much as the first months on immunotherapy may be a draining process for owner and veterinarian, I would consider offering referral to a veterinary dermatologist in selected patients, particularly if you are not experienced in this therapy.

Ectoparasiticidal Agents

When treating patients with ectoparasites, environment and contact animals have to be considered as well. Environmental contamination is always significant with chiggers (*Trombicula alfreduggesi*, *Neotrombicula autumnalis*) typically also with lice and possibly with *Chorioptes* and *Psoroptes* mites. Contact animals must be treated for all these ectoparasites except chiggers. Many ectoparasiticides are classified as insecticides and off-label use is not permitted in many countries.

Insect Control Trials and Individual Management of Patients with *Culicoides* Hypersensitivity

Treatment recommendations will vary significantly with individual situations. Reasonably safe and effective products are available (see Table 3-5). As veterinarians, we are in the best position to advise clients on an insect-control program tailored to their specific needs.

☛ One major reason for failure of insect control programs is owner compliance. They are either unwilling, not educated properly, too careless, or simply not physically able to do what we ask them to do. Choosing the right protocol and educating owners properly will greatly increase your chance of success.

Table 3-5
Selected Ectoparasiticidal Agents in Equine Dermatology

DRUG	FORMULATION	COMMENTS	INDICATIONS	SIDE EFFECTS	DOSE
Ivermectin	10 mg/ml equine oral solution		Effective for *Psoroptes* spp., myiasis, parafilariasis, habronemiasis, onchocerciasis		200-300 mcg/kg q 2 weeks for 4 applications
Lime sulfur	2% solution	Foul odor, stains jewelry and hair.	Effective for nonfollicular mites such as *Chorioptes* and *Psoroptes* spp.	May rarely be irritating	Apply 1-2 x/week for 4 weeks
Fipronil	0.29% spray in 250 ml bottles	Strong smell unavoidable during application.	Spray effective against *Chorioptes* spp. and chiggers	Temporary irritation at site of application	Spray legs from elbows and stifles down.
Pyrethrin	0.06-0.4% spray	Repellent as well as adulticide. Low toxicity potential.	Culicoides hypersensitivity		Spray horse twice daily to weekly
Permethrin		Repellent as well as adulticide. Low toxicity	Culicoides hypersensitivity		Spray horse twice daily to weekly

✓ Stabling during the day (for black fly and horse fly hypersensitivity) or from dusk to dawn (for mosquito and *Culicoides* hypersensitivity) may be helpful.

✓ When stabling the horse, remember that some insects, particularly *Culicoides* gnats, are small (down to 1 mm) and able to pass through normal meshing, so fine meshing is needed to prevent the gnats from entering the stable.

✓ *Culicoides* (in contrast to horse flies or black flies) are weak fliers and a strong fan in the paddock or in the stable blowing against the door or window may be helpful. Alternatively, horses can be moved from sheltered paddocks to areas more exposed to wind.

✓ Environmental measures such as draining marshes or swamps and removing manure or decaying vegetation may be helpful.

✓ Protective covering may be helpful in some horses, particularly if the predominant *Culicoides* species present are dorsal feeders.

✓ Insect repellents such as pyrethrins or pyrethroids may be used daily on the horse.

Immunosuppressive Therapy

💣※ Before you think about immunosuppressive therapy you must be sure about your diagnosis. It can be very dangerous for your patient to start immunosuppressive drugs based only on history and clinical examination, so confirmation of the diagnosis of immune-mediated skin disease is essential. If the horse has an infectious disease (fungal, bacterial, or parasitic), it can rapidly deteriorate. There is no place for trial therapy in immune-mediated disease (!) (except in the case of a patient otherwise facing euthanasia).

✋ Patients with immune-mediated skin disease may have secondary infections that need to be identified and treated initially or concurrently.

🔑 It is impossible to give you a good general purpose recipe for immunosuppression. Every horse reacts differently to each of the drugs mentioned later in this section, and you have to individualize treatment for each patient. Immunosuppression is a technique requiring instinct, sensitivity, and experience as well as theoretic knowledge that is beyond the scope of this text. You may want to consider referral of horses in need of immunosuppressive therapy to a veterinary specialist. There are, however, starting dosages and ranges that can be used as a guide. In horses, non-glucocortocoid drugs are much more expensive treatments than in small animals or humans and often cost-prohibitive, thus typically immunosuppressive therapy will be started with glucocortocoids.

✓ The doses mentioned in Table 3-6 are starting doses that are tapered as soon as possible to the smallest effective dose.

✓ Tapering of a drug commences once the patient is in clinical remission or if adverse effects are intolerable. In a horse with severe adverse effects and concurrent clinical signs of active disease, new drugs need to be added at the same time.

☞ If a well-controlled horse suddenly seems to relapse, always check for bacterial, fungal, or parasitic infections first. Rather than a flare-up of the immune-mediated disease you may be encountering a problem secondary to your treatment. These horses are immunosuppressed and thus may be affected more easily by infectious diseases! Increasing the dose of the immuno-suppressive drug may not be indicated.

Table 3-6
Drugs Used in Immunosuppressive Therapy

DRUG	FORMULATION	COMMENTS	ADVERSE EFFECTS	DOSE	MOITORING
Prednisolone	20-mg, 50-mg tablets, granules	Rapid onset of action, inexpensive, response rate approximately 50%.	Polyuria, polydipsia, lethargy, infections, muscle wasting, laminitis	2 mg/kg q 12-24 h	Clinical monitoring typically sufficient
Azathioprine*	50-mg tablets	Lag period of several weeks. Further reading is recommended before using this drug. Expensive in horses.	Diarrhea (often responding to dose reductions), bone marrow suppression. In dogs, hepatotoxicity occurs and serum biochemistry may be indicated in horses with anorexia	2 mg/kg or 50 mg/m2 q 24 h	Complete blood counts at 0, 1, 2, 4, 8, 12 wk and then every 3-6 mo
Aurothioglucose*	50 mg/ml suspension	Long lag period (6-12 wk). Further reading is recommended before using this drug. Expensive in horses.	Bone marrow suppression, occasional cutaneous eruptions and proteinuria in humans and dogs	1 mg/kg q 7 d IM. Tapering to q 2 wk, 3 wk, 4 wk after remission achieved	Complete blood counts at 0, 1, 2, 4, 8, 12 wk and then every 3-6 mo

Appendix – History Questionnaire

Name:_____ Owner:_____

Breed:_____ Age:_____ Sex:_____

Presenting problem: _____

Pruritus present? ❏ No ❏ Yes If yes, where?

❏ Face ❏ Legs ❏ Trunk ❏ Tail ❏ Dorsum ❏ Neck

❏ Generalized ❏ Permanent ❏ Sporadic

Lesions present?

❏ Excoriations ❏ Crusts ❏ Scales ❏ Hair loss ❏ Hives

❏ Weight loss

Other signs? ❏ Sneezing ❏ Coughing ❏ Eye discharge

When did the problem start?_____

When does the problem occur? ❏ Spring ❏ Summer ❏ Fall
❏ Winter ❏ All year

What leads to deterioration?_____

What improves the problem?_____

Other problems?_____

What do you feed your horse?_____

Are other contact horses affected? ❏ Yes ❏ No Details:_____

Are owners affected? ❏ Yes ❏ No Details:_____

Environment: Inside_____

Outside_____

What do you use for deworming?_____

Fly control measures taken_____

Other medications or supplements: ❏ Shampoos ❏ Sprays

❏ Tablets ❏ Injections

Letzte Tablette gegeben am: __ / __ / __ Effekt:_____

Letzte Injektion gegeben am: __ / __ / __ Effekt:_____

Further comments:_____

Index

Page numbers followed by an *f* indicate a figure; page numbers followed by a *t* indicate a table.

A

Abscess

  Corynebacterium equi in, 59

  diagnosis, treatment, and prognosis of, 56*t*

  treatment of, 72

Acantholytic cells, cytology, 21

Actinic keratosis, 60

Actinomyces, 73*t*

Age, at first clinical signs, 5

Airborne allergies, sneezing and coughing with, 6

Allergen-specific IgE, serum testing for, 34

Allergen-specific immunotherapy, 76

  considerations before beginning, 76-77

  cost of, 77

  duration of, 77

  recommendations in, 77-78

Allergic pruritus, 46

Allergy

  shampoo therapy for, 70, 71*t*

  treatment of, 72

Alopecia

  approach to, 63-67

  with bacterial pyoderma, 52

  biopsy for, 30

  breed predispositions to, 4

  with *Chorioptes equi*, 45

  deep skin scrapings for, 24

  definition, pathogenesis and differential diagnosis of, 14

  in dermatophilosis, 50

  diagnosis, treatment, and prognosis of, 49*t*, 64-65*t*

  duration and progression of, 5

  on face, 51

  with granulomatous disease, 46

  with lice infestation, 45

  linear, 54

  multifocal, 44

  in onchocerciasis, 45

  with pemphigus foliaceus, 52-53

  perineal, 66

  trichogram for, 29

Alopecia areata

  diagnosis, treatment, and prognosis of, 64*t*

  multifocal, 66

Amitriptylline, formulation and dose of, 76*t*

Amyloidosis, 62

  age at onset of, 5

  diagnosis, treatment, and prognosis of, 58*t*

Anagen defluxion, 65*t*

Antibiotics

  dosage and duration of, 72

  indications, formulations/dosages, and adverse effects of, 73*t*

  for nodules, 57*t*

  for papules, scales, and crusting, 48*t*

  response to, 7

Antifungal treatment

  for dermatophytosis, 48*t*

  for nodules, 57*t*

Antihistamines

  advantage of, 75

  for atopic dermatitis, 41*t*

  for pruritus, 75-76

  withdrawal time of, 76

Antiseborrheic shampoo, 48*t*, 49*t*

Appaloosas, predispositions of, 4

Folliculitis, bacterial
  diagnosis, treatment, and
    prognosis of, 48t
  treatment of, 72
Food adverse reaction, 35
Fungal culture
  indications for, 24
  interpretation of, 26-28
  technique in, 25
Fungal infections, 70, 71t
Fungal spores, 29
Fusobacterium, 73t

G

Glucocorticoids
  adverse effects of, 74
  anti-inflammatory dosages of, 77
  demodicosis due to, 65t
  formulation and starting dose
    of, 75t
  for granulomatous disease
    or sarcoidosis, 42t, 49t
  in immunosuppresive therapy, 81
  for nodules, 56t
  for onchocerciasis, 49t
  for pruritus, 41t, 74, 75t
  response to, 7
  for verminous dermatitis, 49t
Glucocorticosteroids, 74, 75t
Gnats, 80
Granulomatous disease
  alopecia and crusting due to, 46
  bacterial, 57t, 72
  diagnosis, treatment, and
    prognosis of, 42t, 49t
  signs of, 6

H

Habronemiasis, 56t
Hair
  color changes in, 9
  fungal culture of, 25

loss of. *See* Alopecia
  shine of, 9
Hair follicle
  dysplasia of, 14
  inflammation of, 14
Haircoat quality, 9
Hematopinus asini, 23, 41t
History questionnaire, 83
Home-made remedies, 8
Hoof, overgrown, 54
Horse fly hypersensitivity, 80
Hydroxyzine, 75
  formulation and dose of, 76t
Hyperadrenocorticism, 72
Hyperplastic dermatitis, 30
Hypersensitivity
  antihistamines for, 76t
  Culicoides, 78-80
  diagnosis, treatment, and
    prognosis of, 41t
  insect-bite, 36
  lesions in, 9
  to penicillin, 73t
  in pruritus, 40
  ruling out, 7
  seasonality of, 6
Hypodermiasis, 56t
Hypotrichosis
  in allergic pruritus, 46
  diagnosis, treatment, and
    prognosis of, 64-65t

I

Imiquimod
  for nodules, 57t
  of occult sarcoid, 64t
Immune-mediated dermatoses, 72
Immune-mediated skin disease
  age at onset of, 5
  crusting in, 47
  lesions in, 9

Organophosphate rinse
for mange, 42t, 49t
for pediculosis, 41t
Otitis externa, 42t

P

Papular dermatosis, 4
Papules
approach to, 47-55
in coital exanthema, 54
deep skin scrapings for, 24
definition, pathogenesis and differential diagnosis of, 11
diagnosis, treatment, and prognosis of, 41t
with insect bite hypersensitivity, 43
trichogram for, 29
Paraffin oil, in superficial skin scrapings, 22
Parafilaria multipapulosa, 56t
Parafilariasis, 56t
Pediculosis, 41t
Pelodera strongyloides, 49t
Pemphigus foliaceus
age at onset of, 5
alopecia and scaling with, 52-53
contracted heel and overgrown hoof in, 54
crusting with, 47
cytologic diagnosis of, 21
diagnosis, treatment, and prognosis of, 48t
Penicillin G, 73t
Penicillin V, 73t
Permethrin, 79t
Phaeohyphomycosis, 57t
Pigmentation change, 10
Plaques, 11
Poxvirus, 49t
Prednisolone
formulation, adverse effects, and dose of, 82t

formulation and starting dose of, 75t
for pruritus, 74, 75t
Pruritus
alopecia with, 63, 67
antihistamines for, 75-76
approach to, 40-46
diagnosis of, 41-42t
differential diagnosis of, 41-42t
duration and progression of, 5
glucocorticoids for, 74, 75t
identification of, 5-6
key questions for, 40
with nibbling of distal limbs, 44
prognosis for, 41-42t
serum testing for, 34
severity of, 6
shampoo therapy for, 71t
superficial skin scrapings for, 22
treatment options for, 41-42t
Pseudomonas aeruginosa, 73t
Pseudomycetoma
diagnosis, treatment, and prognosis of, 57t
lesions of, 9
Psoroptes
superficial skin scrapings for, 22, 23
treatment of, 78
Psoroptes equi, 42t, 49t
Psoroptes hippotis, 42t
Psoroptic mange
age at onset of, 5
duration and progression of, 5
Pulmonary edema, 6
Punch biopsy, 31-33
Purpura hemorrhagica, 6
Pustules
definition, pathogenesis and differential diagnosis of, 11
remnants of, 15
trichogram for, 29

Pyoderma
  crusting and alopecia with, 52
  treatment of, 72
Pyrethrin
  formulations, indications, side
    effects and doses of, 79t
  for insect hypersensitivity, 80
  for mange, 42t, 49t
Pyrethroid
  for insect hypersensitivity, 80
  for mange, 42t, 49t
  for pediculosis, 41t
Pythiosis, 58t
Pythium insidiosum, 58t

Q
Quarter horses, predispositions
  of, 4, 5

R
"Railroad-track" appearance, 21

S
Sabouraud's agar, 25
Salicylic acid shampoo, 71t
Saprophyte culture, 26
Sarcoid
  diagnosis, treatment, and
    prognosis of, 57t, 64t
  flat, 67
  nodules, crusts, and ulceration
    due to, 60
  occult, 64t
  verrucous, 61
Sarcoidosis, 42t, 49t
Sarcoptes, 23
Scabies
  duration and progression of, 5
  superficial skin scrapings for, 22
Scales
  approach to, 47-55

definition, pathogenesis and
  differential diagnosis of, 14
fungal culture of, 25
with pemphigus foliaceus, 52-53
skin scrapings and cytology for, 55
superficial skin scrapings for, 22
Seasonality, 6
Seborrhea
  diagnosis, treatment, and
    prognosis of, 42t, 48t, 49t
  scaling and crusting with, 47
  shampoo therapy for, 70, 71t
Seborrhea sicca, 71t
Seborrheic dermatitis, 71t
Self-trauma, 14
Serum testing, 34
Shampoo therapy, 70, 71t
  failure of, 70
  indications for, 71t
Skin, inspection of, 10
Skin disease
  breed predisposition to, 4-5
  duration and progression of, 5
  seasonality of, 6
Skin scrapings
  butter the bread motion in, 17, 18
  for cytology, 17
  deep, 24
  for scaling and crusting, 55
  superficial
    indications for, 22
    interpretation of, 23
    technique in, 22-23
Skin surface cytology. *See Cytology*
Spongiosis, 12
Sporothrix schenkii, 57t
Sporotrichosis, 57t
Squamous cell carcinoma
  diagnosis, treatment, and
    prognosis of, 57t
  on penis, 60

NOTES

NOTES